D0721663

Tantric Orgasm for Women

Diana Richardson

Destiny Books
Rochester, Vermont

Destiny Books
One Park Street
Rochester, Vermont 05767
www.InnerTraditions.com

Destiny Books is a division of Inner Traditions International

Library of Congress Cataloging-in-Publication Data
Richardson, Diana.
  Tantric orgasm for women / Diana Richardson.
      p. cm.
  Includes bibliographical references.
  ISBN 0-89281-133-1
  1. Sex instruction for women. 2. Female orgasm. 3. Sex—Religious aspects—Tantrism. I. Title.
  HQ46.R465 2004
  613.9'6—dc22

                                                            2004003673

Printed and bound in the United States at Lake Book Manufacturing, Inc.

10 9 8 7 6 5 4 3 2 1

This book was typeset in Garamond and Weiss, with Medici Script and Avant Garde as display typefaces

All Osho quotes printed with permission of Osho International
Artwork prepared by Alfredo Hernando, Madrid, Spain.

Dedicated to Love in Women

Contents

Acknowledgments

I sincerely thank the many women who have shared their experiences with me over the years, and from whom I have learned an inestimable amount. In particular I am grateful to the women who have given me permission to use their personal words of experience, which have helped enormously in conveying the true map of female sexuality, and thereby of love. In addition, I am thankful to the male partners of those same women, because their mutual experiences in love made this direct contribution possible. I have also included a few sharings by men and I am grateful to them for giving me permission to do so. I vouch for the absolute authenticity of all the personal experiences I have quoted. I have, for simplicity's sake, elected not to identify the individual contributors by name or initial.

Introduction

In Sanskrit, the ancient religious and classical literary language of India, the word *tantra* can be likened to such concepts as "capacity for expansion" and "that which goes on expanding," and the words *continuum, web, context,* and *transformation.*[1] Tantra teaches an acceptance of who we are as a whole, from the solid density of our physical body to the refined layers of our spirit. It is concerned with the transmutation of energy, liberation of the mind, attainment of one's full potential. The balanced union of opposites is considered the way of achieving liberation of mind and body, a liberation from the supposedly endless cycle of unconscious rebirth. Tantra understood over five thousand years ago what modern science has since proven to be true through chromosome study: that woman is half man and man is half woman. The balancing of inner opposites is the way to achieve full potential. Falling fully into feminine mode in sexual union transforms woman through an inner alchemical process.

This, my second book on tantra, essentially explores tantra from the female perspective. In the pages ahead I endeavor to convey the significant role that receptive feminine energy plays in the male-female sexual exchange. It wouldn't be realistic to draw a distinct line between woman and man when talking about sex because sex is the most intimate meeting of the male and female elements. However, there are aspects of sexuality that apply exclusively to women, and these can be used to distinct advantage in influencing and strengthening the sexual experience—for both women and men. A woman who is without a partner can still benefit from this knowledge. It can give her a new feeling about herself and her body, and often through this new awareness she will draw the right partner to herself.

As a researcher, teacher, and writer on sex, I have been encouraged by both women and men to address sexuality from the female point of view. Women have suggested this directly; and though no men have exactly verbalized it, I have been encouraged indirectly by men's actions and what they have demonstrated, unknowingly, to me in the last twenty years.

In this time many couples have attended the "Making Love" workshops for couples that I colead with my partner, Raja. During the workshops, truly touching miracles take place every day. Many of the couples reexperience the dynamic love that brought them together in the first place, and have been able to continue into the future in loving harmony. However, not all partnerships are equally successful and sometimes couples have separated. In time, naturally, those who have separated have formed new relationships. As these new relationships begin to take hold, I've noticed something quite phenomenal and unexpected happening in the groups. The men who had attended my workshops before are returning to the workshops. It is the *men* who have been coming back to share this alternative approach to sexuality with their new female partners because they have experienced how the tantric approach can enhance love. To my greatest surprise, women (though they found the first workshops as uplifting as their partners did) have been much slower on the rebound. Only in the very recent past have women participants come back to repeat the workshop with new loved ones.

The fact that many men but few women return to the workshops with their new lovers offers two important insights. The first is that we women are afraid to talk to men about sex and are reluctant to share with men what pleases our bodies most. We hesitate to introduce our male partners to any alternative sexual approaches. The main fear for a woman is that of losing her man, of ceasing to be sexually attractive to him if she changes. Sadly, when women choose to stay with conventional sex—which is a distorted form of male sexuality—we give away our unique feminine magic and power.

The second insight is much more encouraging, and I hope it will give women the confidence to be more authoritative in the sexual sphere. The fact that men *are* bringing women back to the workshops clearly demonstrates that men develop a liking for another form of sexual expression once they have tasted it. How can a man have a taste for something he has never experienced? Often tantric sexuality has to be experienced before the longing for it can arise.

From both men and women who have no personal experience with tantra I repeatedly hear the comment, "Tantra seems to be for women, not for men." Based on my own exploration and on the encouraging response of the men who attend my workshops, I can say with all certainty, "No, tantra is not only for women. It is definitely for men too." Tantra is not simply something designed to make women happy (and men not so happy), a way of giving women the reins for a while. When a man has had one taste of the delicious depths and heights of expanded sexual energy, invariably he wants it again. But unless women make available their true femininity to men, how and where and when can men develop a taste for it?

Here and there you might find a woman who naturally has the knack of receiving and channeling masculine sexual energy upward during intercourse and can lift sex to another dimension for herself and her man. The truth is that a woman can consciously develop this art and guide her man into an expanded sexual sphere—and thereby create for herself more satisfying sexual experiences. A woman has the natural capacity to enter this realm simply by virtue of being a woman. She who is the receptive aspect in the male-female dynamic can move inward and draw or pull man along with her. This is her intrinsic power. Through receptivity, through giving way and yielding, inherent movement is possible. The opposite does not hold quite so true: generally speaking, man cannot easily initiate the experience of opening a doorway and absorbing woman into him. To do so requires great stillness and the clarity of true male authority. When the receptive (feminine) aspect gives way, actually receiving what is coming to it, its very receptivity enables the dynamic (masculine) energy to move and flow. In this way man easily and naturally follows woman; he can even wordlessly flow into exalted realms with woman *if* he is fortunate enough to encounter receptive feminine energy.

Woman is the real starting point for the necessary reeducation in sex. This movement has to take root in women and spread from them out into society—through lovers, friends, one-night stands, through mothers teaching daughters and fathers teaching sons. It requires that women begin to speak up for themselves, expressing their needs and sensitivities, and that men take urgent heed of these messages. The greatest potential for true sexual fulfillment and love lies in a woman and a man joined together on a mutual journey of sexual self-discovery.

Nevertheless, a woman can do much without the conscious cooperation of a man. Sex is about as close to ourselves as we can get; it reaches, touches, and changes every cell of our bodies. Through exploring sex we will discover who we really are beneath all the social pretensions and conventions that we habitually use to cover up our deeper sexual selves.

My source of tantric inspiration and guidance is my spiritual master, Osho. Osho, or Bhagwan Shree Rajneesh, as he was known earlier in his life, teaches meditation not as a practice but as a way of life. He is a mystic who brings the timeless wisdom of the East to bear upon the urgent questions facing men and women today. He speaks of the search for harmony, wholeness, and love that lies at the core of all religious and spiritual traditions, illuminating the essence of Christianity, Hassidism, Buddhism, Sufism, Tantra, Tao, Yoga, and Zen.

There are no words to express my depth of gratitude for his profound and continuing impact on my life. Osho's interpretation of the ancient tantric scriptures creates a superior body of knowledge and insight that I have been fortunate enough to have access to since my mid-twenties.

Tantra is beyond technique; it is a profound journey of self-discovery and self-transformation, an alchemical process of transmuting base energies to higher spiritual expression. Some techniques can be used along the way, but the secret of tantra lies in bringing that which is sexually unconscious in us into full consciousness. Osho says, "Tantra is the transformation of sex into love through awareness." This implies that *how* we do something is infinitely more important than *what* we do.

It is my privilege to include some excerpts of Osho's tantric inspiration throughout this book. It may perhaps interest the reader to know that Osho's words, appearing here in text form, were initially delivered as off-the-cuff oral discourses, completely spontaneous and without any previous preparation, at gatherings for his disciples and interested public in India. Later these were published in book form. I wish to make it clear that the handful of quotes appearing here are simply those that I chose to include. They in no way represent the full range and extraordinary diversity of Osho's spiritual insight into the human condition.

Osho Speaks on Sex

I have almost four hundred books in my name. Out of four hundred books there is only one book on sex, and that too is not really on sex; it is basically on how to transcend sex, how to bring the energy of sex to a sublimated state, because it is our basic energy. It can produce life. . . . It is only man who has the privilege to change the character and the quality of sexual energy. The name of the book is *From Sex to Superconsciousness*—but nobody talks about superconsciousness. The book is about superconsciousness; sex is only to be the beginning, where everybody is.

There are methods that can start the energy moving upwards, and in the East, for at least ten thousand years, there has developed a special science, Tantra. There is no parallel in the West of such a science. For ten thousand years people have experimented with how sexual energy can become your spirituality, how your sexuality can become your spirituality. It is proved beyond doubt—thousands of people have gone through the transformation. Tantra seems to be the science that is, sooner or later, going to be accepted in the whole world, because people are suffering from all kinds of perversions. That's why they go on talking about sex as if that is my work, as if twenty-four hours a day I am talking about sex. Their repressed sexuality is the problem. My whole effort has been how to make your sex a natural, accepted phenomenon, so there is no repression—and then you don't need any pornography; so that there is no repression—and then you don't dream of sex. Then the energy can be transformed.

There are valid methods available through which the same energy that brings life to the world can bring a new life to you. That was the whole theme of the book. But nobody bothered about the theme, nobody bothered about why I have spoken on it. Just the word *sex* was in the title, and that was enough.

The book is not for sex; it is the only book in the whole existence against sex, but strange. . . . The book says that there is a way to go beyond sex, you can transcend sex—that's the meaning of "from sex to superconsciousness." You are at the stage of sex while you should be at the stage of superconsciousness. And the route is simple: sex just has to be part of your religious life, it has to be something sacred. Sex has to be something not obscene, not pornographic, not condemned, not repressed but immensely respected, because we are born out of it. It is our very life source. And to condemn the life source is to condemn everything. Sex has to be raised higher and higher to its ultimate peak. And that ultimate peak is samadhi, superconsciousness.

Osho, transcribed teachings,
Sex Matters: From Sex to Superconsciousness
(included at the request of Osho International)

1

The Intrinsic Potential for Orgasm

*E*ach and every woman arrives on this earth with the intrinsic capacity to experience the uplifting joy of orgasm. Mother Nature in her unswerving wisdom has graced the female body with a special design so that this experience can arise. Women have the potential to live sex fully, as a conscious, guiding force. However, even though nature may have sincerely intended this for us, in real life very few women can say that they have genuine command over their orgasmic experiences. Instead, for most women, orgasm remains quite elusive, happening now and then, depending more on good orchestration than on an intimate understanding of our inner design. Love becomes an experience filled with ups and downs: it doesn't seem to last long enough; is as changeable as the wind; is one day here and gone the next. Women living without the ambience of love suffer tremendously, often experiencing states of acute depression and despair.

In part this unhappy situation can be attributed to a lack of insight into feminine energy and the female body. Women have no information on how to intentionally create the orgasmic state or how to embrace the gift of orgasm. In this void of wisdom, woman does not understand herself as intimately or expertly as she could. As a consequence, this naiveté about her body operates unconsciously against her better interests—in life, in love, and in sex.

Recently, at the end of a couples workshop, a man participating with his wife summed up his experience to the group: "It is quite incredible. After spending the last thirty-five years trying to become a really good lover, I discovered during this week that everything I think turns a woman on in actual fact turns her off." His observation was correct. I too have observed that the opposite of almost everything people think or say about sex has proved to be the truth. As a result of these misconceptions, women on the whole are not at all satisfied with the state of their sex lives, finding them unfulfilling for any number of reasons. Perhaps this may not be so at the beginning of a sexual relationship, but after a period of time many women report that dissatisfaction has become the norm. The body gradually closes down and a general disinterest and disappointment in sex begins to creep in. For some women this shift can occur within a few months, for others it happens over the course of a few years. The length of time involved is not relevant; what is most significant is the fact that this withdrawal from sex happens repeatedly for women.

Not knowing her body and the "how" of expanding into her feminine energy automatically places a restriction and limitation on a woman's experience of sex, and therefore of love. And if this reality is true for woman, it is equally true for man. If woman is living and loving at a sexual minimum, her male partner also exists at this same level.

For women this sexual minimum is reflected in their tremendous difficulties at achieving orgasm. So often women share with me their fear that something is seriously wrong with them because they cannot manage to experience any kind of orgasm. Or they're worried because they need an hour or more to feel a full *yes* to penetration. Or they report that sex has gradually lost its attraction, though the longing for tenderness and intimacy remains. With these negative thoughts passing through the mind, old and unexpressed feelings of unworthiness or inadequacy can ripple to the surface; soon insecurity begins to erode the joy of a loving heart. For a woman, unhappiness and dissatisfaction with sex can easily become the acceptable, expectable norm. Women's magazines routinely give tips on sex and female orgasm and advice about how to achieve orgasm more easily. Simply because these articles speak openly about sex (a rare occurrence in everyday conversation), they might gratify and relax a woman for a short while. But the guidance these magazines offer barely scratches the surface of the deeper sexual realm that exists for every human being. The advice found in magazines also reflects the widespread absence of concrete information on the female body. When last did we hear anything new or inspiring? When did we last hear about something that works? something that sounds right or feels right? something that resonates in the body, heart, and soul?

The truth is that your body is fully capable of experiencing deep, rich, satisfying orgasm. The key is to step inward and observe the physical sensations of your own body without judgment. How do you feel when you are having sex with your partner? How do you feel when you are having sex by yourself? Gather information about your body's responses. What do you enjoy? What irritates you? What leaves you feeling profoundly disappointed? Remember that, as long as you look at them honestly, feelings are always true. No feeling is ever "wrong."

When your partner, consumed by excitement, begins to move ever harder and faster toward his own climax (the so-called jackhammer mode), do you feel invisible, left behind, engulfed by a wave of disappointment that once again he will be all finished before you even begin to get warmed up? Or perhaps your partner dutifully feels that he should satisfy you before he allows himself to be satisfied, so he works hard to bring you to orgasm by stimulating your clitoris. He's doing the "right" thing, so you don't want to be critical. But is he rubbing too hard? too fast? Do you need more lubrication? Do you feel pressured to get on with it, to hurry up and climax so that he can move on to the "real" part of sex—that is, penetration and ejaculation? Do you worry that he's getting bored while he's stimulating you? Do you find yourself getting bored? Do you leave your body altogether and make a grocery list in your head or remember that your second child needs to take a picnic lunch for his field trip tomorrow? Or do you need to leave your physical body in another way and engage in a steamy sexual fantasy in order to come to climax? Do you actually feel disinterested but work hard at that fantasy, nevertheless, because your partner will be disappointed or feel diminished if he can't bring you to orgasm? Do you sometimes fake orgasm just to get the whole thing over with?

You are not alone. Unfortunately, most women in our modern-day cultures have felt some or all of these ways. And all of these scenarios miss the essential truth that your body is fully capable of a deep, sustained, fully satisfying orgasmic state. Orgasm is not a destination that we arrive at by trying—by doing the right thing or thinking the right thoughts. Rather, orgasm is a state of being that arises naturally when we are more relaxed in sex. In relaxation woman opens to her inner world, bringing herself into the focus of her attention. Doing so reveals the exquisite interplay of active male and receptive female energy, which flowers into prolonged pleasure for both the man and the woman.

You may well ask, "If this is true why don't more people know about it? Why has sexual dissatisfaction become the rule for women, rather than the exception?"

It can be said that we human beings unconsciously remain short-sighted about our true sexual selves. We are unaware of our higher potential and how to access it. As it stands, in our conventional sexual expression we are not truly physically sensitive or psychologically receptive or available enough to invite higher sexual experiences into us—or rather, to be graced by the divine, which would be a more accurate description. We are as host, and the divine is as guest, and enormous space has to be created for the divine to enter us.

These days it has become virtually impossible to shine new light on sex, to look at it and see it in a fresh, innocent, enlightened way. This is because there is an inherent limitation in our viewing situation—woman's role in the sex act is always looked at through the same spectacles, through the prevailing misconceptions about sex, the very misunderstandings that lie at the root of the orgasm issue. If you were to always look at the world through rose-tinted lenses you would begin to believe that everything was pink. If no one ever suggested that you take your spectacles off and see how the world looked without them, you might continue to believe in your rose-tinted perceptions. They would become the norm for you, just as our misconceptions about female sexuality have become the norm for us in today's world.

Take, for instance, the sometimes-proffered suggestion that a woman use sexual fantasy to provoke an orgasm. In actual fact, sexual fantasy has nothing to do with what is happening in the woman's physical body in the here and now, with this particular man. It is an imagined scenario. It is a deliberate switch over from channel "body" to channel "mind," using the power granted by imagination. This can in fact trigger the response of sexual excitement in the body. But it has nothing to do with the physical penis that is present right now in the physical vagina. The issue here is that basic to lack of orgasm is a lack of connection to the body and to its internal sensitivity, its kinesthetic sense. So the advice of fantasy as a solution to orgasm—which only absents a woman further from her physical body—keeps woman circling around in the same sexual frame in which she already finds herself.

Our conventional, socially conditioned view of sex is linear and one-dimensional, lacking in balance, intelligence, and spiritual insight. Unless we are taught the full potential of sex while we are young, we inherit a sexual conditioning just by being a part of our society, by being surrounded by cultural misinformation that we absorb unconsciously. The rare person is able to access the uplifting dimension of sex intuitively; most of us are conditioned and live life in innocence of any sexual alternatives.

In response to the unconscious female conditioning of our society, the essential female qualities often become distorted: Softness can become weakness; receptivity can become passivity or resignation; the nurturing quality can become overbearing; the beauty of surrender can become submission; absorption might turn into sucking; the ability to sustain long-term waiting can shift into indolence; love can turn to jealousy and the use of female qualities for manipulation; the joy of non-doing and relaxation can express itself as the dead weight of inertia and laziness. Feminine fluidity might become a state of collapse; the free expression of individual feelings shifts toward sentimentality or moodiness; intuition and psychic abilities can slide over the line into paranoia and hysteria; the ability to allow events to unfold without trying to control them can become inappropriate indecisiveness or lack of initiative; sensitivity twists into victimhood or is used in the service of fear; appreciation for beauty becomes attachment to outer appearance; the nesting impulse can become a compulsive obsession with security; silent strength can turn to masochistic dependency; the awareness of connection to the universe beyond one's personal boundaries can go too far, resulting in an individual who is vague and spaced out and lacking enough personal definition.

The currently accepted view of "normal" sexual experience keeps women in bondage to an expression of a male type of sexuality, with no room for expression of the equally important female pole of sexual experience. The current male-oriented approach features an outward, sensation-directed expression of sexuality that effectively erases intrinsic female qualities, and in so doing firmly plants the roots of sexual dissatisfaction and dysfunction in both sexes. It is exactly the feminine, receptive qualities (undistorted by cultural misinformation) that are absolutely essential for the orgasmic state to arise in woman and also in man. Woman is required to be physically more poised and at ease so as to absorb the true male force, transform it, and channel it upward through her receptive feminine powers.

At this point in time women unconsciously, and sometimes consciously, support men in their male-oriented expression of sexuality. Many women report a high incidence of pain during and after sexual intercourse, but they endure it silently in order to satisfy their partners. Many others assume that sex will be a rough, aggressive experience with no expression of love or tenderness. I remember a woman telling me during a workshop that she had no idea that sex could be considerate and gentle. We collude with the dominant form of sexual expression simply because lovemaking has been "done" in this way for as long as we can remember. By now it seems utterly normal and we are unaware that alternatives exist.

While it appears that the conventional model of lovemaking is more satisfying for men than for women, in truth men's sexual fulfillment could also be much fuller and deeper, more sustained and more satisfying than it is now. One reason for this is that male ejaculation is commonly understood to be the male version of orgasm. For many men ejaculation *is* the sexual experience. However, ejaculation is not the equivalent of orgasm. There is another type of male orgasm that happens without ejaculation and release of semen, an orgasm in which the energy is retained in the body, expanding upward instead of being released outward.

Women have enormous difficulties in reaching any kind of satisfying orgasm, while ironically (and yet somehow not surprisingly), men face the completely opposite problem—orgasm (or at any rate, ejaculation) is uncontrollable. It is impossible to delay or avoid. Usually it happens immediately upon penetration (or shortly before), or else within a paltry few minutes. The amount of time that passes between penetration and ejaculation is way too short for the purpose of raising a woman's sexual temperature to a sufficiently high degree that she will experience orgasm.

Once a woman discovers the art of expressing herself within the female element, with more serenity and receptivity, she will find to her surprise that she automatically reduces the likelihood of her man ejaculating prematurely. In this way, woman has the power to extend lovemaking from minutes into hours. A perceptive, sensitive internal environment can be consciously created by a woman. This environment changes the whole quality of the exchange and has the added power of strengthening the true masculine response. Distressing male sexual problems such as impotence and premature ejaculation are also symptoms of the prevailing confusion and lack of information about sex, and particularly about the female body. When woman develops the ability to shift into her feminine nature, exercising her receptive powers, many of these sexual dysfunctions and dissatisfactions can be healed.

At first most women will feel that they have little idea of how to shift into their feminine aspect or what that truly means. In reality it is easy—and it is absolutely natural. When we connect with our feminine qualities we can truly be who we are, with nothing forced and nothing acted out, we are simply open to receiving love. Relaxation, innocence, grace, and loving spontaneity are at the core of femininity. Women in my workshops frequently describe the shift toward themselves as a "coming home" to something they have always known intuitively. Some share with me the sadness of recognizing now, so many years after their first glimpse of the truth, the insufficient trust they have had in themselves to follow through on their intuition and bring it into experience.

Feminine wisdom is nature's jewel, held deep within woman. The pages ahead are an attempt to help women uncover something they already possess, a crystal waiting to receive the light of inner intelligence.

Tantric Inspiration

Energy can have two dimensions. One is motivated, going somewhere, a goal somewhere, this moment is only a means and the goal is going to be achieved somewhere else. This is one dimension of your energy, this is the dimension of activity, goal oriented—then everything is a means, somehow it has to be done and you have to reach the goal, then you will relax. But for this type of energy the goal never comes because this type of energy goes on changing every present moment into a means for something else, into the future. The goal always remains on the horizon. You go on running, but the distance remains the same.

No, there is another dimension of energy: that dimension is unmotivated celebration. The goal is here, now; the goal is not somewhere else. In fact, you are the goal. In fact there is no other fulfillment than that of this moment—consider the lilies. When you are the goal and when the goal is not in the future, when there is nothing to be achieved, rather you are just celebrating it, then you have already achieved it, it is there. This is relaxation, unmotivated energy.

OSHO, TRANSCRIBED TEACHINGS,
TANTRA: THE SUPREME UNDERSTANDING

Awareness and Sensitivity Preparation
Position for Rest and Relaxation

Here is the ideal horizontal position to assume for relaxation: Your head, neck, and spine should be in a straight line, not even a few millimeters out of alignment and definitely not with the head rolled away to one side. Your legs should be straight and a little apart, and your ankles should *not* be crossed over each other. Place a narrow soft pillow (or a rolled blanket) directly under the knees to create a slight curving and softening of the knee joint. Place a small, flat, firm pillow (or folded towel) under your head. Pull the chin to the chest so as to straighten your neck before placing the pillow in position. The pillow should support the lengthening of your spine so there is not too much of a curve in the neck. If the chin is pointing almost directly upward and not tilted toward the chest, use a slightly thicker pillow (or give the towel another fold) to lift the head an additional few inches, so as to create length and reduce the curve in the neck. Place your open hands palm down on the groin area on each side of your pubic bone. Rest quietly with closed eyes for twenty minutes (or more), holding awareness in your body.

Tantric Meditation
Growing in Consciousness

Lying in the position described above, you can deepen your experience if you close your eyes and imagine yourself looking into your body. Imagine that your eyes can look inward and downward into your body, even as far as your genitals. Breathe deeply and slowly into your belly, as if the breath is massaging your insides and touching the genitals. Continually pull your attention back into your body and the sensations in it. Deliberately disconnect from distracting thoughts when they pop up. Let them float away, and return to your body. Immerse yourself in the body so that you feel a sense of resting deep within your body, with the sensation of being submerged in yourself.

Travel with your awareness to any places in the body where tinglings or warmth or fine vibrations are present, and dissolve into them.

At a certain point, once the practice of immersing into your senses takes root, the feeling of your physical boundaries will disappear; you may experience being as light as a feather, bathed in golden light, floating suspended in consciousness. You are, but you are not. In this way you can grow in consciousness until every cell is penetrated. The moment consciousness touches the cells, they are different. The very quality of the cells changes.

You can set a clock for the period of time you wish to devote to the experience, or you may leave it up to your inner clock, which, after a period, spontaneously returns you to normal consciousness (along with the sense of having lost all track of time). You are likely to notice that after such an experience you feel refreshed and rejuvenated, as though you have had a drink directly from the source of life. It is also beneficial to practice this meditation before sleeping at night, or at any time during the day when you need to recharge your energy.

2

Orgasm Is a Spiritual Experience

Probably most of us have given little thought to where the word *orgasm* comes from, and what it actually implies. *Orgasm* derives from the Latin word *orgia*,[1] which describes a pagan religious ceremony in which people became ecstatic—so ecstatic that their bodies were bursting with divine energy and they were able to lose themselves in time-stopping bliss. In the word *orgasm* we see our origins reflected in language, reminding us that in earlier days humans gathered together in large groups to perform rituals with the intention of deliberately moving into ecstasy. Attaining orgia was a way of praising and expressing gratitude to Mother Earth, extolling the marvel of her creation. With simple dance steps, singing to the rhythmic beating of the drum, and celebrating for days on end people became almost drunk with the divine, accessing gloriously heightened states of sensuality and sensitivity. Participants returned from the ceremonies rejuvenated, overflowing with love and zest for life.

Today few opportunities for expression of orgia exist. There has been a shift away from emphasis on the physical body toward emphasis on the mind. Instead of sharing energy by dancing and singing together, people are more likely to meet in large or small groups to exchange ideas, discuss, argue, or gossip. We have become disconnected from our bodily sensitivity and lukewarm in our physical responses; as a result we experience a lack of fulfilling orgasm during sexual exchange. In this restricted environment sex loses its natural healing and regenerative powers. Man and woman have lost touch with the uplifting spiritual connection once regularly accessed through the physical body.

Human beings can only genuinely begin to affect or change their social environment through a dramatic and drastic reevaluation and re-evolution in sex. The repression and suppression of normal, healthy sex that has prevailed for the last few thousand years of civilization has had a severely polluting effect on the beautiful, loving, natural expression that sex is. At present it can safely be said that the source of most social disturbance and violence has its root in sex—or, more to the point, the lack of nourishing, fulfilling, uplifting sex. It is as if our society has become sexually unwell. Sex itself is not sick, but the mind—the psychology of humans surrounding sex—has become tainted, almost toxic. The sexual abuse of all kinds that occurs somewhere every minute of every day provides acutely painful evidence of the sexual distress present in society. Through widespread misinformation, sexual energy is unconsciously repressed and creativity is diminished. The prevalent lack of understanding about the nature of male and female energetic interaction means that contemporary sex rarely achieves a full expression of its spiritually regenerative potential. Although at first glance sexual perversion, sexual abuse, aggression, and war might not appear to be directly related to a lack of fulfilling and nourishing sexual experience, the rejection of an expression that is our inherent nature contributes to all of these unfortunate outcomes.

Through misunderstanding the significance of sex over and above reproduction, a woman can easily find herself forced to accept a loveless, intrusive, and abusive sex life. She may sincerely want to produce children and to love, feed, and care for a family, yet she devotes herself to all of this heartfelt expression in the absence of any regenerative and uplifting orgasmic experiences for herself. And this lack of sexual fulfillment holds true for men, too, most of whom, even after a lifetime of sexual experiences, still believe that ejaculation equals orgasm (which, as we have already mentioned, it does not).

Biology, as the means by which life here on Earth is preserved, is without question basic to sex. Without biological sex, life as we know it would cease. Almost all forms of animal and plant life unite male and female elements to re-create life. Sometimes the two elements are in separate entities, sometimes not. Sometimes the entities join physically, sometimes not. In whatever way the miracle of fertilization occurs, sex functions to create new life, extending the collective life of all the species. Sex fully engages all levels of life in all forms in a most extraordinarily wholehearted process in order to ensure the continuation of the species.

Even though it is no novelty, human birth will forever be the most awesome of miracles. The innocence, integrity, and delicate perfection of translucent new life touches and warms the heart in the most enchanting of ways. Even so, the ability to reproduce another human being represents only our basic biological expression of sex. This is our so-called animal nature, and it depends upon a downward movement of energy. Male semen is released by ejaculation (with or without female orgasm). Fusion and fertilization of the female egg follows, and another life is initiated, a life separate from the two lives that produced it.

But there is more to human sexuality than the physical ability to reproduce. Nature did not give us the captivating mystery of sex simply for quick male ejaculation and prolonged female gestation. In humans there is a higher dimension to sex—there is more to the meeting of male and female than meets the eye.

The Upward Movement of Sexual Energy

Humans are designed to experience altered states of consciousness during sexual union—states that engender a blissful experience of union with the whole of existence. In this orgasmic ability we differ from our friends in the animal kingdom (with the exception of dolphins, who are understood to experience higher energetic states during sexual play). Our bodies come with the innate capacity to expand energetically from the sexual center. When correctly harnessed this expansion results in altered states of consciousness: valleys of ecstatic relaxation and peaks of orgasmic expression.

The impact of upward-moving sexual energy is relatively unknown in the West and is explored by only a few. But if we turn to the East we encounter (in China) a far earlier culture whose medical practitioners urged such energy practices for good health and longevity. In India a far earlier religion also recognized and cultivated this upward-spiraling energy as the spiritual aspect of sex, as sacred sexuality.* When the energy is routed in this vertical way as an expression of the higher, generative aspect of sexuality, sex protects the body and is experienced as a rejuvenating and life-giving force in the human being.

In generative sexual expression, the intent and function are more or less opposite from the intent and function of its biological counterpart. There is no biological requirement to ejaculate semen (to coincide with ovulation). No additional life is produced; instead, the energy is retained and remains within the participants themselves, renewing lives that already exist. The lovers feel enriched, energized, loving, and joyful.

Inward and upward movement of energy during generative sexual play occurs of its own accord with the balance and alignment of male and female genitals. Energy moves according to an innate polarity, which we discuss in depth in Chapter 4. Genitals together generate energy that rises upward through internal channels eventually to reach, and return to, the "master" endocrine glands in the brain, the ultimate source of all hormonal information given to the body.

These glands, particulary the pituitary and pineal glands, themselves produce our sexual expression.[2] (At high levels of hormonal purification, the body will even release perfumed fragrances.) The pituitary gland is

---

*China (Taoism), three thousand years ago and India (Tantra), five to ten thousand years ago.

located between the eyebrows, above the nasal cavity. It is the master endocrine control gland regulating growth, gonadal function, the adrenals, and the thyroid. This gland is said to govern the forebrain, vision, and the right eye, as well as being the seat of love, compassion, knowledge, love of humanity, and devotion. It is also involved in intelligence and conceptual memory, which we use in reading, thinking, and studying. Close by is the pineal gland, located toward the crown of the head above the midbrain; its functions are related to sensitivity and to the sexual cycle. The pineal gland governs the hindbrain, hearing, body rhythms, equilibrium, and the perception of light through eyes and skin.

Given all of these functions that we take for granted, it becomes obvious that feeding and nourishing these master glands with our sexual energy—our life force—is bound to be to our distinct advantage.

When energy spirals upward it produces a vitality that radiates from the whole being. One feels cellularly drenched with contentment, love, and peace. Sex experienced in this way is empowering. Energy is not released; it is produced, strengthening the immune system and enhancing all kinds of creativity. An individual can extend her life by producing this generative energy rather than simply duplicating it, as is possible through the downward-moving expression of reproduction. Nature gives us sex so that we may have the opportunity to transcend the limits of our physical boundaries, to float as filaments of vibrating light and love. The experience of generative sex keeps a person youthful, adventurous, and responsive to whatever life brings.

It seems incredible to realize that the spiritual realm of orgasm—the most fulfilling gift human beings possess—remains unexplored during an age in which humankind has penetrated outer realms with its increasingly sophisticated technology. In spite of all of our technological know-how, we find ourselves stumbling around in the sexual arena, tethered by ignorance and by complacency. We assume that simply by virtue of being a woman or a man, we will automatically know everything about the sex act.

How then is it that woman knows so little about her body and her sexual potential? Perhaps at some time in the past this knowledge was deliberately kept secret from her, making her a more compliant slave to the appeasement of mans' appetites. But it comes as no surprise to women that modern men are even less informed than women about women's bodies—or, for that matter, about their own bodies. Women have a longstanding affinity with intuitive knowledge—commonly referred to as "women's intuition"—which most men are less able to access as the truth residing within their bodies. By looking (and feeling) within, women need to take the lead in making a place for generative sexuality, and for the love that follows.

In the absence of a woman's cooperation in sex, the divinity of the sex act is near impossible to encounter. Generations of insensitive handling and abuse of women by men has led to situations in which sex, to a lesser or greater degree, is lovelessly imposed upon women. When a man repeatedly enters a woman's body before she is really prepared for penetration, the woman will feel turned off to sex. A certain repulsion may even begin to set in. In time, many a woman will close down physically, eventually turning away from sex if possible. When unable to avoid it, she becomes a master at submitting, enduring the minutes prior to ejaculation. Once she becomes resigned to lack of satisfaction in sex, woman can actually feel grateful for premature ejaculation in the knowledge that everything will soon be over.

Man has lost his masculine ability to "speak" meaningfully to the female body, the ability to spiral in on her in such a way that she welcomes penetration with her whole being. He has become so accustomed to woman giving in and yielding to him that he has forgotten (or has never experienced) the true taste and flair of cooperative sexual expression, the dance of male and female sexuality in perfect balance, in which woman sumptuously participates, transforming the experience into a sinuous, winding, dynamic dance between bodies. Such an experience in itself can give man the feeling of his worth as a male of the species—and for many a man it will be the first time he feels this way in his life.

Woman Is the Environment of Sex

It is impossible for man to know more about a woman's body until she comes to know a little bit more about herself. With constructive input, a woman can learn how to transform the quality of her sexual experience, even in the absence of conscious cooperation from her man. Woman's influence in the sexual realm is such that she can drastically alter the experience *if* she knows how. This gives her the capacity to make satisfying love for the rest of her life and to find the love she seeks without necessarily having to change partners.

Because a woman's body is most often judged from the outside by its shape, its proportions, and its curves, a woman has a bird's-eye view of herself. She is accustomed to seeing herself from a distance, from without; rarely does she truly feel herself from within. When a woman learns how to nourish a romance with her own body, to unite with it from the inside, alive in all her senses, she exudes a breathtakingly feminine quality that transforms the atmosphere around her.

Unfortunately, most modern women have no information whatsoever on how to accomplish such a transformation. Out of disappointment and frustration, many women today abandon sex altogether, trusting that their love for children or career will compensate for the loss. In so doing a woman commits a travesty of justice: she denies herself an essential part of being a woman. Resignation begins to settle firmly around her mouth. Often a woman feels a longing for grandchildren (for another cycle of reproduction) so that she may once again feel love flowing within her.

In an ideal world, grandmothers would inspire their grandchildren by talking freely about their most nourishing experiences with sex, guiding their grandchildren along the right track, encouraging them to give and receive love. But as it stands in our culture, our mothers and grandmothers and great-grandmothers have, like ourselves, had no access to higher forms of sexual expression. In the sexual realm, they have nothing to pass down in the way of wisdom or insight.

This does not mean that no such wisdom exists. When we look to ancient traditional cultures of the East we find an open conduit to sexual wisdom. Central to that wisdom is the knowledge that woman is the environment, the container, the receptacle for sex. Her vagina is the space into which man physically *enters*. And, in great contrast, woman *receives* man physically into herself. These two functions—entering and receiving—are very different. Man is the guest; woman is the host.

Because of the internal design of the vagina, woman is able to exert a powerful influence during the sex act. This command that a woman has in sex, as the environment of sex, can best be illustrated by simple analogy. If you were to enter a room that was crowded with furniture and hectic with the blaring sounds of a television and the ringing demands of a telephone, this atmosphere would likely have a negative impact upon you. It would probably strike you as being frenzied, congested, chaotic, and a bit overwhelming. You might feel encapsulated by pressure and tension, and most likely your immediate impulse would be to get out into the open air again as soon as possible.

In contrast, if you were to enter a room that had a feeling of spacious emptiness enhanced by just a few essential furnishings, where the sound of a flute hung suspended in air that was fragrant with sensuality, such an environment would exude peace and tranquillity. Rather than inspiring tension, it would inspire a sensation of inner space, expansion, a feeling of coming home. The embracing atmosphere, the absence of external pressures, and the open space would give rise to an inner relaxation. As harmony and serenity descended upon you, you would probably take a deep breath and arrive fully in your body.

Now consider the event of male penetration into the female body. Just as the environment in a room has a profound effect upon the human psyche, the ambience within the female body can, and does, have a transforming effect upon man. It is extremely influential. Man is utterly affected by woman and yet he is ignorant of the extent to which this is so. Through intentionally creating a serene, receptive internal environment a woman can prolong the sex act. She can help man to delay, and even to avoid, ejaculation.

The real sadness, though, is that woman remains as unaware of her true capacity as man does. Not knowing how to tap into it, she too fails to experience her intrinsic power, leaving her deeper realms of female sexuality unexplored. Understanding the real nature of female sexual expression can reunite woman with her god- and goddess-given power. When woman enters the sexual act within her female element, sexual fulfillment and love will be the natural consequence. Every woman possesses this natural ability to transform lovemaking into a wholly satisfying and spiritually transcendent experience. All women need is useful information on how to go about it.

Tantric Inspiration

Orgasm is a state where your body is no more felt as matter; it vibrates like energy, electricity. It vibrates so deeply, from the very foundation, that you completely forget that it is a material thing. It becomes an electric phenomenon—and it is an electric phenomenon.

Now physicists say that there is no matter, that all matter is only appearance; deep down, that which exists is electricity, not matter. In orgasm, you come to this deepest layer of your body where matter no more exists, just energy waves; you become a dancing energy, vibrating. No more any boundaries to you—pulsating, but no more substantial. And your beloved also pulsates.

And by and by, if they love each other and they surrender to each other, they surrender to this moment of pulsation, of vibration, of being energy, and they are not scared. . . . Because it is deathlike when the body loses boundaries, when the body becomes like a vaporous thing, when the body evaporates substantially and only energy is left, a very subtle rhythm, but you find yourself as if you are not. Only in deep love can one move into it. Love is like death: you die as far your material image is concerned, you die as far as you think you are a body; you die as a body and you evolve as energy, vital energy.

And when the wife and the husband, or the lovers, or the partners, start vibrating in a rhythm, the beats of their hearts and bodies come together, it becomes a harmony—then orgasm happens, then they are two no more. That is the symbol of yin and yang; yin moving into yang, yang moving into yin; the man moving into the woman, the woman moving into the man.

Now they are a circle, and they vibrate together, they pulsate together. Their hearts are no longer separate, their beats are no longer separate; they have become a melody, a harmony. It is the greatest music possible; all other musics are just faint things compared to it, shadow things compared to it.

OSHO, TRANSCRIBED TEACHINGS,
TANTRA: THE SUPREME UNDERSTANDING

Awareness and Sensitivity Preparation
Developing Soft Vision

To help your energy (which usually moves outward) to fall back in upon your own heart, it is helpful to learn *soft vision*. In soft vision you reverse the usual visual process and imagine you are receiving inwardly through the eyes rather than looking out through them.

To begin: stand, sit, or lie (in the position described at the end of chapter 1). Close your eyes and bring awareness to your body, finding a location such as the belly or heart or solar plexus that feels like "home" to you. It should be a place that easily connects you to your inner world and acts as an anchor for your awareness in the body. It is a resting place, an inner resource around which you gather yourself and from which you experience and create the present moment. If your whole body feels like home to you and there is no specific area that grabs your attention, a generalized body awareness is fine too.

When you have the sense of being rooted in your body, connected with yourself from the inside, open your eyes extremely slowly, millimeter by millimeter, allowing anything that falls into your range of vision *into* yourself *through* your eyes. It can be a flower, a candle, a plant, a painting, a view in the room, a wall, a ceiling: simply imagine that whatever appears before you—the texture, the light, the color—is *entering* you, penetrating you through your eyes. The looking becomes passive, as if vision is reversed. Your eyes are receiving energy, not dispersing energy, as seems to be the case in normal looking.

While practicing this way of seeing, the trick is to pay attention to your body and to stay rooted in the bodily home you have identified. The intention is not to lose the connection to yourself once your eyes are opened. Losing connection to the body when the eyes are open is bound to happen again and again as you make your first few attempts. As soon as you notice you are absent from your body, more involved in looking outward than directing your awareness to your inner world, close your eyes immediately and reconnect inwardly for several seconds. When settled and rooted inside again, open the eyes very slowly. Continue with this process of opening the eyes while staying connected to the body and closing when you lose connection until you get the hang of it. Practice is required in the beginning; after a while it will become easy. You can also practice soft vision in nature—with a waterfall, with a tree, with a sunset, with the moon—and you will have memorable experiences of peace and love.

Tantric Meditation
Meditating on Light

When you feel comfortable with soft vision you can make a special meditation of it using the power of light. Meditation on light is one of the most ancient meditations. Light has been emphasized because meditating on light causes something inside you that has remained asleep to start opening its petals. Through time and the collective wisdom of those seeking transcendence through the body, this process has come to be associated with the light-sensitive pituitary gland, situated in the body at the site of what yogis call the third eye.

Give yourself half an hour or more for this experience. Create a harmonious environment and sit in front of a candle. Using soft vision, allow the flame to enter you. When the eyes need a rest or you lose connection to your body, close your eyes and continue to visualize the light penetrating you through your eyes. Alternatively open and close the eyes as feels most comfortable to you.

Let light become your meditation: whenever you have time, close your eyes and visualize light. Wherever you see light, be in tune with it, be alert to it, be prayerful toward it, be grateful to it.

3

Orgasm versus Orgasmic

The nature of female orgasm is not easily generalized—quite possibly there are as many kinds of orgasm as there are women having them. Even so, in order to understand the nature of feminine energy it is helpful to look at orgasm from a number of angles.

Orgasm can be loosely divided into two categories—peak orgasm and valley orgasm. Naturally there can be a whole range of experiences between a peak and a valley, but what distinguishes one from the other is the very basis of each type—the peak orgasm depends on an active buildup of excitement and the valley orgasm arises from relaxation.

Peak and Valley Orgasms

Let us consider in detail the differences in these two approaches to orgasm. From the very outset the approach and attitude is different, one from the other. First of all, we tend to intentionally seek and "go for" the peak type of orgasm, to deliberately build it up to a climax. Achieving a peak orgasm becomes a linear, goal-oriented activity requiring a mental intention to get from one place to another. We assume that we need to *do* whatever we consider necessary to reach our final destination—the peak. A valley experience is more like an invitation without an expectation or demand of orgasm. Something may or may not happen. And when it happens, it happens by itself. The final outcome is not at issue; rather, the focus is on the joy of the moment—being here and now in the body—which allows the journey to unfold without a predetermined direction. In place of pursuing an orgasm there is an openness to and acceptance of what is taking place in the body, moment by moment, which creates the sensitivity necessary for an orgasmic valley experience to emerge.

To arrive at a peak orgasm we must usually expend considerable physical effort. The aim is to intensify the stimulation and bring the deliciously exciting sensations into one glorious crescendo. This involves repeated mechanical movements of the pelvis, which get faster and faster toward the end. This activity is necessary in order to intensify energy to a peak, but at the same time it also builds up a lot of tension, which compresses the energy into the genitals. In contrast to all this customary activity, to enable a valley experience to flower we need to *be* more and *do* less, allowing everything to unfold very slowly in the most languid, easy, lazy way possible. We avoid deliberate efforts and any movements or positions that produce undue tensions. The penetration of the vagina by the penis is deliberately slow, and so are any pelvic movements. This relaxation between the genitals encourages a radiation and expansion of energy into other parts of the body.

The peak orgasm is usually quite a hot affair. In the valley things are a lot cooler. Any pleasurable moments of excitation can be enjoyed for what they are, but they will be followed by minutes of relaxation, not fed and inflamed into a climax of excitement. Through slowing down into a more non-doing approach and bringing awareness to internal movements of energy, we awaken an inner sensitivity that has little to do with excitement or stimulation. This sensitivity reveals a layer of magnetic excitation in the body that is cool, cellular, and ecstatic. A buildup of excitement is not even really required for the relaxed kind of orgasm.

Yet another way that a peak orgasm differs from a valley orgasm is in the duration of the experience. A peak orgasm is estimated to last, on a good day, around ten seconds. So we can say that a peak experience has a pretty definite start and finish. This makes it more like an event—we "have an orgasm," or not, as the case may be. In contrast, the valley orgasm is a more sustained state, a timeless experience without a specific start or finish. It can last for a few moments or a few hours—the time span is irrelevant, but the experience is the same: In a valley orgasm, an ecstatic peace descends upon us, it surrounds, embraces, and soothes us, we are suspended in it. We "become orgasmic." This is an expanded state of consciousness, not a momentary event measurable in seconds, like an orgasm.

When we merge fully with the subtleties present in the physical body, the sexual experience becomes ecstatically bodiless. This sounds contrary and upside down but in reality this is how it works. Energy turns inward and expands, streaming orgasmically upward. Rather than being discharged or released from the body, the energy gathers within the system, generating vitality and creativity. Sex experienced in this way enhances and strengthens the life force: beneficial hormones released during sex are delivered to the brain, nourishing the master pituitary and pineal glands situated there (as mentioned in the last chapter), with positive impact on good spirits, health, and longevity. Sex actually extends life.

The energy of a peak orgasm tends to work in the opposite way. In the peak experience the energy moves downward and outward, in accordance with the requirements of procreation. The intensity of excitement is followed by a pleasurable discharge of energy that is released down and out of the body. Evidence of this discharge is the fact that frequently after ejaculation a man will suffer a distinct loss of energy. He may even feel angry, restless, or disconnected from his woman. Many women observe that they too lose great amounts of energy in orgasm, just like a man but without the release of semen. Suddenly the willingness to make love evaporates; they find themselves without energy or inclination to continue. As a result of the discharge in an orgasm, a woman can often feel abandoned, lonely, sad, or depressed.

The peak orgasm is more or less experienced as a local genital experience because the sexual energy is not given the chance to expand, to touch other parts of the body. In fact it cannot expand because the very effort of achieving orgasm creates tension and thus a barrier to radiation of energy. The potentially beneficial energy is lost in release, rendering it unavailable for performing its natural healing and nourishing functions.

Special techniques do exist for deliberately extending the peak type of orgasm into multiple orgasms. By synchronizing breath and movement and relaxation, it is possible to assist energy to move beyond the automatic barriers and create expanded energetic states. Reaching these states usually requires substantial skill and focused concentration; rarely, though, do extended peak orgasms arise from an original state of relaxation.

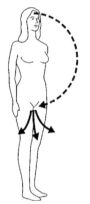

Fig. 3.1. Biological or reproductive phase of sexual energy

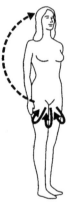

Fig. 3.2. Spiritual or generative phase of sexual energy

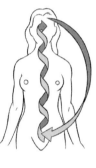

Fig. 3.3. Complete sexual energy circle with redirected sexual energy spiraling through energy centers

Opening to a New Approach

To make the sexual experience more fulfilling, in general, a woman would do well to tend toward the orgasmic approach—orgasm as a sustained state of being in the sexual exchange—rather than simply seeking out the peak type of orgasm. This approach depends a lot on the willingness to trust relaxation and intrinsic feminine receptivity. Rather than trying to make something happen, you simply receive, and *be,* and absorb energy into the core of the body through the vagina. It's natural once you get the hang of it. All the same elements of sex are present but the composition is entirely different. What makes the greatest difference is the attitude and awareness of a woman within herself, a woman's willingness to tap into her true feminine spirit. This requires a deeper understanding of her body and the courage to honor and express the feminine element residing within.

Most women associate the clitoris with orgasm; however, the vagina is more centrally associated with orgasmic states. A rising understanding of this may lead a woman to reevaluate her clitoral experiences while exploring her orgasmic potential. (Chapters 6 and 7 are devoted to the vagina and the clitoris respectively.) Please be aware that when I suggest this alternative approach to orgasm my intention is to broaden the possibilities for satisfying sexual experience. It is *not* my intention to make you think in duality, to suggest that you make a separation between peaks and valleys or doing and being. In reality one cannot exist without the other, so any separation between them is false. Included are all the delightful gradations of exploration and experience linking these two. My intention is to convey that there are choices.

I simply invite you to reflect on your experience in light of the new information I offer here, to see how it might be of benefit to you. With this new approach, the orientation is toward relaxing into being orgasmic rather than searching with effort for an orgasm. Please don't be judgmental toward yourself for your "failure" to have orgasms or for having the "wrong" kind of orgasm. There is no wrong or right way to approach sex, no one to please but yourself. Perhaps, upon reflection, you will realize that you haven't allowed yourself to turn inward during sex, to feel yourself on the inside and discover what would please you. Perhaps you'll see that you've been working awfully hard to *succeed* at sex, as though you were performing in a play or taking an examination. Perhaps you'll conclude that you're basically happy with your sex life but the idea of trying a new approach appeals to your adventurous spirit. It is my sincere hope that whatever insights you gain about yourself by looking inward can shift your perspective in a way that allows you to improve your experience.

Relaxation and Tension

Relaxation lies at the very base of any enhancement of experience, so relaxation and more satisfying orgasm go hand in hand. All orgasms, peak and valley, are enhanced by relaxation. Any relaxation (even briefly) of any body part invites the expansion of energy on which all orgasm and heightened experiences are based. Relaxation spontaneously leads to increased awareness, bodily sensitivity, and psychological openness. And relaxation produces qualities essential to feminine energy. Especially for woman at first, relaxation is essential because it shifts her away from the active, outward, male kind of expression required for conventional orgasm and puts her unquestionably into the receptive, feminine mode. An orgasmic state, or any orgasm achieved through relaxation, engages the genuine, deep-rooted, feminine energies of a woman, which allow orgasm to be a fully satisfying experience. This is a good point to remember when you feel unsure about branching out and exploring a new approach to sex.

Peak orgasms can certainly feel wonderful in themselves, but rarely are they deeply moving. We often feel basically untouched by them. If you find yourself reluctant to explore something other than the tried and true, remember that there is more to sex than the candles on the cake, which can be blown out at any moment. Remember, too, that countless women report problems with the conventional peak style of orgasm, with getting their candles blown out nicely. Even with every best intention, it is not always possible to build up sufficient sexual charge to produce a meaningful or prolonged climax. In our effort to "get there," our movements become faster and harder, more and more unconscious and aggressive, decreasing our sensitivity with each move we make.

The physical tensions inherent in the goal-oriented approach to peak orgasm are compounded by mental and emotional concerns about orgasm that are present even before we begin to have sex. Tensions increase with any kind of pressure and, unfortunately, most women feel pressured to have an orgasm in order to please the man. Man so enjoys the moments when a woman orgasms that he likes to make it happen if he can. Partly he likes to give his woman pleasure, but beyond that the ego issue is a very big part of the picture. When a man sees his woman orgasm, it confirms to him that he is indeed a good lover. This is something for a woman to be aware of, and we'll attend to it more in a later chapter. It is good to know that many men are quite identified with (even addicted to) the excitement of their woman's orgasm, if she is so lucky as to have one.

I am reminded of an occasion in a workshop when, after a few days of experimenting, a woman joyfully announced that she was finished with regular orgasms. They did not really do anything for her. In fact, she even noticed she felt much better without them. (I have heard women say words to this effect more times than I can count.) Much to her surprise this woman's lover took her words very personally and reacted by withdrawing into angered silence. He unfortunately managed to receive her experiential observation as a personal insult—a message that he was no good and had been unable to satisfy her in the first place. He also felt threatened by the possibility that she would no longer be willing to have sex in the usual way, to try for peak orgasms for him or with him. Apparently he would have to sacrifice his customary approach.

Overcoming a Lover's Resistance

Be prepared for a little protesting from your man here and there, but don't let that stall you for long. Don't be too serious in exploring new sexual pathways; develop a sense of humor. Be a sincere adventurer rather than a giver of rules and regulations, a tendency that women can easily display when entering this new realm. Don't get caught up in telling a man what to do and how to do it. The tantric realm is closer to woman because of her receptive nature, so she falls into it more naturally. Man has quite some dismantling of a huge, excitement-oriented sexuality to do. He requires understanding, even compassion; instead of criticizing him a woman can become a bridge for him, a way to cross back and forth between the new and the old approaches. For a man to become tantric requires the same inward focus as it does for a woman, in order for him to contact his natural masculine responsive force and not depend on the usual male strategies. Give him space to experiment, working in cooperation with the reality (man's sexual conditioning) without getting fixated on the ideal, which will only cause tension and turn an adventure into a struggle. Of course, many men are delighted when women take more of a commanding role in sex. Thus your man may welcome your new interest with relief, and not see it as a threat to his ego. Certainly the situation has most potential when you explore together rather than as two separate persons each intent on his or her own thing.

Nevertheless, a woman can try out many of the suggestions offered in this book without her man necessarily having to agree (although he is bound to notice there is something more enchanting about the experience of making love with her). The truth is, changing a style of making love is an individual commitment, not necessarily a couple commitment. You as an individual have to wish to be more aware, receptive, and open—not too dependent on what your partner is up to or expects of you. Otherwise you can go around in circles and never break out of the trap you find yourself in.

For example, the situation may arise that your man wants to come. What do you do? You might join him, saying to yourself, "Well then, what the heck, so will I." But this is not individual commitment; this is handing over to another person the responsibility for your own transformation. And that never works to one's greatest satisfaction. Instead you might choose to *not* come, to relax and enjoy being with him during his experience but not force yourself into coming just because he is doing so. And if you decide, in fact, that this time you do want to come, then set about it in an easier and less effortful way. Be experimental and create the opportunity to experience yourself differently. Resist falling back to the known you, the tried and tested way. Experiment for your own sake and be curious about the outcome.

It might happen that, for a period of time while making love, a man still insists on his orgasm. But in the new context this can be after *an hour of delicious lovemaking*—which greatly changes the picture. And why not? In time, he may feel that it is less important to ejaculate, that he is pretty happy with how things stand at the moment; he feels quite fulfilled and notices he is energized afterward. Through experimenting and observing the outcomes of sex, sex begins to gain significance beyond simple entertainment. This is our usual gauge of sex—did we have fun? Was it recreational? In actual fact, far more telling about whether a good time was had or not is what happens *after* the experience.

Observe the Afterward

We tend to overlook how we experience ourselves after the sexual encounter. How do we feel? What is happening within me and between us? In workshops I insist to couples that "the time afterward is your teacher," not my partner and I. By keeping an eye on your postcoital states, both of you will get insights into the genuine goodness of sex and what leads you where. If after making love there is at times a feeling of distance and at other times a feeling of closeness, what does this reflect? Review your lovemaking and see how it informs you. In time a totally new vision of sex starts to emerge through understanding your experience. The inquiry becomes, "How is sex able to spread its benefit to every moment of my life, every day, in and out of bed? How do I get the best out of sex as a human being, not just a human doing?"

Recently I received an email from a couple in Australia that may serve to relax women and encourage men. After they had found a section of my first book displayed on the Internet, the male partner wrote to me saying:

> We printed the lot and took it away with us on our January break. The simple concept of letting go of goal oriented intimacy has been a revelation which has greatly enhanced the spiritual sensitivity of our lovemaking and the sheer pleasure and beauty of enjoying each moment for itself, the beauty of the feelings of each touch or caress, the moment by moment sensation of each kiss, the loveliness of each moment of body contact, instead of each action being part of the path to the goal of orgasm. Being prepared to throw away the goals and letting each moment lead to the next brings pleasure to each moment and takes away all pressure to perform. We have been married almost twenty-five years and the spiritual dimension has always been important to us, but it is easy to get caught up in our Western approach of being goal oriented in almost everything we do, and so much of the Western material we read about sex is goal oriented. Best Regards.

Open up to the new alternative way, so that your man too can begin to experience himself in a new way. Remember, it takes a morsel before the taste can develop. Don't just give in to going with the usual, the male-dominated sexual expression. A real woman does not stand a chance there. In giving in (or giving up), both men and women are the losers and nobody is a real winner.

Orgasm is a gift from the divine, a sip of the sweetest nectar. It is nothing to demand, expect, or chase after. If there is too much tension coming from expectations in sex, misery or frustration is bound to follow failure. Orgasms are not required every time we make love. An easygoing, innocent, unexpectant attitude creates the milieu for the orgasmic experience. So begin to change your thoughts on orgasm. As you enter sex, do something unusual: forget about orgasm. Avoid looking for sensations that could be the beginning of a climax; avoid heading for orgasm the moment your man penetrates you. Be as receptive and welcoming to the penetration as possible, paying close attention to the feelings in your vagina.

Observe within yourself the minute cellular phenomena present in the body in any given moment. As time is comprised of millions of magical moments strung together, the details are constantly changing, and these can become a constant source of delight.

Living these inner changes makes the sexual experience an organic one. Orgasm is not necessarily a huge explosion, a volcanic eruption. It can be a cool, peaceful, calm, relaxing valley where the body floats as light as a feather, dissolving into love-drenched nothingness. It can be the experience of eternity, beyond time, suspended in space by breath, one with the pulsation of life. It also happens, as if by miracle, that from this depth of relaxation a peak of energy arises, but without any effort at all. A subtle force rises slowly and steadily from the depths and moves into a sexual dance, choreographed by a divine energy passing through the bodies.

Tantric Inspiration

Relaxation is a state. You cannot force it. You simply drop all negativities, the hindrances and, it comes, it bubbles up by itself. What is relaxation? It is a state of affairs where your energy is not moving anywhere, not in the future, not to the past—it is simply there with you. In the silent pool of your own energy, in the warmth of it, you are enveloped. *This* moment is all. There is no other moment. Time stops—then there is relaxation. If time is there, there is no relaxation. Simply, the clock stops; there is no time. This moment is all. Relaxation means this moment is more than enough, more than can be asked or expected. Nothing to ask, more than enough, more than you can desire—then the energy never moves anywhere. It becomes a placid pool. In your own energy, you dissolve. This moment is relaxation. Relaxation is neither of the body nor of the mind, relaxation is of the total.

OSHO, TRANSCRIBED TEACHINGS,
TANTRA: THE SUPREME UNDERSTANDING

Awareness and Sensitivity Exercise
Partner Exercise to Harmonize the Energies

An energy-harmonizing exercise such as this one can be used to attune you and your partner to one another. Give yourselves about half an hour. It can be done as described here, as a practice in itself, or as a mode of foreplay that continues into making love. The harmonizing exercise finishes with both of you standing up, which is really one of the best ways to begin making love—kissing and embracing and gradually proceeding to the bed.

Prepare a meditative atmosphere around you and your partner. Place cushions opposite each other a little distance apart. (Use chairs if necessary.) Sit upright with crossed legs, if possible, and a comfortably straight spine. Your spine will be better supported if you sit directly on the bones of the buttocks (sitz bones), so do lean forward and pull the flesh of your buttocks slightly apart and away from you. This will create a slight arch in the lower back, which makes sitting on the floor with crossed legs easier to sustain.

Sit facing each other in the night, by candlelight or by moonlight, and hold each other's hands crosswise. Use soft vision, as described at the end of chapter 2. For about ten minutes look into one another's eyes; if your body starts swaying, allow it to. You can blink, but go on looking into one another's eyes. Whatever happens, don't let go of one another's hands. After ten minutes, close your eyes and allow the swaying to continue for a further ten minutes.

Then stand and sway together, holding hands for ten more minutes. You can have eyes open or closed, whatever feels most comfortable for you. Finish with a warm embrace. This exchange will mix your energy deeply.

4

The Source of Orgasmic States

$\mathcal{T}$here are many reasons why the sexual exchange often does not lead to orgasm for women. One of these reasons is that the sex act is much too short, due to the chronic premature ejaculation that exists among men. A few minutes of sexual intercourse does not remotely begin to tap the orgasmic energies of a woman. The most important reason, though, is that the *real source of female orgasm is misunderstood.* We require concrete information about the delicately designed energy that exists in the female body. Orgasm should be a relatively effortless affair. Ecstasy is our natural state: we are all born ecstatic, but sadly, throughout childhood we slowly lose access to our ecstasy in becoming socially conditioned. Still, we are made for ecstasy and it can be relearned.

Equal and Opposite Forces

Too easily we assume that the energetic bodies of man and woman are in effect the same. In reality a woman's body is completely different from that of a man's and exactly to what extent our bodies differ has not been understood. Any differences between us are taken for granted, while the deeper implications are missed.

If we look at the differences that are apparent between male and female bodies—the sexual organs and associated reproductive functions—what can we see? We see the unique male ability to produce and discharge seeds containing half the blueprint for life. We see the unique female ability to receive, absorb, supply the other half of the blueprint and transform it into life within her. Reproduction demonstrates that male and female are equal forces in perfect balance: one no stronger, one no weaker; each providing a vital function. Man cannot reproduce himself on this planet without woman, and woman cannot create life in the absence of man. These two equal forces are absolutely opposite in expression while at the same time utterly complementary. There is an active force balanced by a receptive force.

Woman's body is equal to man's body while simultaneously energetically opposed to it. So, in sex, what goes for a man (apparently) is not *necessarily* energetically suitable or true for a woman. In being opposite and equal to man, woman complements man in his entirety. This equal and opposite phenomenon underpins the powerful pull of sex—we are continually drawn to the opposite sex regardless of our age and it seems that sex will not leave us in peace, or at least not for very long. Actually, sex is knocking on our door, offering a secret way to attain profound peace and love through male and female elements being rightly harnessed. By meeting, melting, and merging with the opposite force, we become complete, we become one. The sense of separation evaporates into the sense of immense union with everything that is. Most people in our societies today hold sex and spiritually far apart, and many even consider them to conflict with one another. Yet the longing for union (with the opposite sex or with existence itself) is a spiritual longing, which reveals why, in their essence, sex and spirituality are so closely associated.

Energetic Differences of Woman Compared with Man

We hear little about different energetic qualities of female and male and a lot about constitutional and emotional differences. A basic education should include a study of how our different energies manifest in our physical differences—and what significance these have in the sexual exchange. Nature intentionally instilled the female and male genitals with complementary qualities, or polarities of energy, in order that they might interact and play with each other.

The female element is receptive and the male element is active.* Many other words can be assigned to describe these essentially opposing qualities, such as yin/yang, moon/sun, night/day, passive/dynamic. The meeting of female and male is a meeting of opposite poles, and this meeting makes a flow of energy possible between them. At the subtle energy level this complementary design produces, with relative ease, an orgasmic state. By virtue of *not being the same*, these equal but opposite forces create one vibrant unit. Only when these two halves meet is the sexual unit complete. Imagine a lock and key. A lock without a key is basically useless. A key without a lock is equally as useless. Together, through one fitting into the other, they perform an essential function. Even though each part is quite different in design, when the fit is true the unit rotates and a secret door swings open to reveal a paradise of hitherto unknown sexual experience.

In addition to the existence of this polarity, we must understand that woman is in fact half man and man is half woman. It is this inner phenomenon that forms the basis of meditation. It is helpful to use the magnet as a model to understand more fully our internal design. Although the human body is not absolutely identical to a magnet, it is similar enough to make the magnet model useful in perceiving the body energy in a different way. Poles of a magnet are traditionally assigned "positive" and "negative" to convey their essential attributes. Overall a woman is negative and receptive, but within herself she carries the equal and opposite pole of experience. In accordance with her receptive nature, the vagina, which receives man physically, is the negative pole. The opposite pole, the male pole, exists in the breasts and heart. All the male attributes and qualities—such as dynamic, active, sun, yang—then apply to the positive pole, the breasts/heart of the woman. From here she opens, radiates, expands, expresses, shares, reaches out into the world. However, through the vagina

---

*Please note the important difference between action and activity as explained by Osho in chapter 9. Action comes out of a silent mind; it is a true response to a present situation. Activity is an irrelevant pouring out of restlessness carried over from the past.

she serenely welcomes, sweetly receives, absorbs, and relaxes. Woman as passive aspect represents the negative pole, yet within herself she carries the positive.

Furthermore, between opposite poles there is a flow of energy. A channel of what can best be called electromagnetic energy, known in tantra as the *magnetic rod,* runs between the lower and upper poles of the female body. Between positive and negative is a movement of subtle electromagnetic energy that streams or spirals and becomes the source of the orgasmic experience. The ultimate source of orgasmic experience lies *within* each individual, not outside.

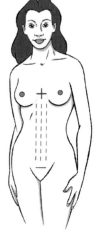
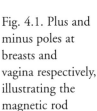

Fig. 4.1. Plus and minus poles at breasts and vagina respectively, illustrating the magnetic rod

Orgasm Is an Auto-Ecstatic Phenomenon

This means that essentially orgasm is an auto-ecstatic phenomenon that comes to pass through the interplay of equal and opposite polarities. Woman embodies the feminine passive principle externally, yet internally her male aspect balances this. In woman, the outer feminine pole triggers the activation of the inner male pole, opening a channel to the streaming of orgasmic electromagnetic energy.

Interestingly, the genital contact of the penis in the vagina is not absolutely essential for an orgasmic experience. The human being is auto-ecstatic: given the right environment, it is possible for anyone to move into states of ecstasy alone. Anyone can be blessed with an experience of ecstatic bliss *without* sexual intercourse.

In reality, then, another person is not involved in your ecstasy. It may be triggered by your partner in making love, but the inner experience, the ecstasy and joy, is yours alone. The person may or may not share a similar experience, depending on his presence and sensitivity. For instance, a woman can have an ecstatic sexual experience even while a man is fast asleep inside her without erection. In sex we are engaging with the other, having the source of orgasmic energy triggered, yet ultimately the state is experienced as our own. It is not always mutually experienced as the same thing at the same time.

Blissfulness requires only three essential elements: timelessness, egolessness, and naturalness.[1] The beauty and elegance of sex is that these three essential elements are naturally made possible by the sexual situation itself. Tracking backward and recovering our innocent, natural, egoless selves in sex, we shift into a realm where time dissolves and bliss descends.

A woman shares her experience: "I had a very strong experience of the energy field beyond the bodies, watching the bodies inside the energy space. The weird thing was that this was all happening while my partner was in total misery and couldn't feel any of it. Is this possible? It reminded me of similar experiences I've had before, lying on top of a man with him still inside me, me not moving, in bliss and joy and then the man would start snoring—he was not there with it at all (consciously at least), and then I always thought I must be imagining the bliss and energy, and I would cut it off immediately."

Two Magnets Meeting at Opposite Ends

While women are essentially auto-ecstatic, we can engage with men to galvanize our inner opposite into life—to awaken us to our inner source of ecstasy. It follows then that the male body, equal and opposite, will have the magnetic poles reversed. The positive pole is the penis, in accordance with the physical design for penetration of the vagina, and the negative pole is the heart and chest. As in woman, between these two poles there is an electromagnetic streaming, an ecstatic flow of energy. In relation to woman the male "magnet" is standing on its head in a

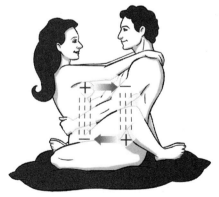

Fig. 4.2. Opposing female and male polarities, with magnetic rods and potential circular energy flow (in "yab yum" position)

reversed position. When a man stands *opposite* a woman, their inner magnets are meeting at their opposite ends—negative vagina to positive penis and positive breasts to negative chest. This is why some people avoid close hugs except with their intimate partner, and even there I see many couples keeping their pelvises withdrawn from a full-body embrace, simply out of a lifetime of habit. We avoid touch or pressure between the genitals or breasts and chest because a powerful polarity exists, and the connection is sometimes not appropriate when hugging friends or strangers.

When opposite poles are facing one another and brought into proximity, two magnets will exert a tremendously attractive force on one another. (On the other hand, magnets with similar poles facing will repel one another and push apart.) When two magnets meet at opposite poles the magnetic field is tremendously amplified. In fact, the magnetic field is then much larger and more intense than the sum of its two parts.

The attraction of magnets is due to a circulation of electromagnetic energy that is created between the two magnets, with plus flowing to minus (man to woman) and plus flowing to minus (woman to man) at both ends. Woman recirculates energy received in the vagina by channeling it upward and radiating out through her breasts to man, as the positive flows to negative. Man radiates from the penis into woman and correspondingly receives from woman through his heart. There is a reciprocal circle, a circling force of energy.

Allow Physical Contact to Be Porous

Couples will feel the power and attraction of this phenomenon when standing opposite each other, even at a distance of a yard or two apart. Some couples find it even easier to feel the energy circling from a distance than when they are in physical contact. As they get physically closer other distractions get in the way, perhaps fears of being truly open or fears of not being accepted fully, or perhaps the physical contact will be so compact as to deaden the finer sensations in the energy field between the bodies. For this reason, *porous* contact is always recommended when bodies are up against each other, as in an embrace. Bodies need to contact each other extremely delicately; otherwise, finer sensations easily get overshadowed. When a man squeezes you firmly in his arms during an embrace, you will not be able to stay in his arms for very long. After a few moments, there comes an urgent need to pull back into your own space because it is too physical, too hard, and the sensation of being hugged is not that enjoyable, not after the initial joy of the greeting and kiss. There must be a quality of porousness wherein a person respects your energy body, which extends way out beyond your physical boundaries. In the porous situation a hug can be sustained for hours as the energy bodies melt deeper and deeper into one another. Usually during physical contact we don't think about a person's energy body, but we all have one, although some of us are more aware of it and sensitive to it than others.

When we become more sensitive to ourselves and to our partner, we begin to perceive the true communion between man and woman. Man gives to woman as positive force and woman receives from man as negative force. In her very receiving she is empowered and returns that power by giving to man, and thus he receives what he himself has given. In giving, man receives and in receiving, woman gives. When he knows how to speak to the body of a woman through polarity, the love a man gives returns to him through his woman. It is recorded that an actual circle of light can start to move between a couple, and they will begin to emanate light. This is an interesting image to have as inspiration; however, reaching such heights requires much preparation and loving patience.

The Circling of Love Energy

The energy circle as an image can help you. With practice and in good time, this circle may be an outcome, but it can never be a goal. When a man is able to experience his woman as his equal and opposite, love is created in her and returned to him through breasts and heart. The second part of the magnetic circle is complete. The inner magnets and outer magnets are in accord. This unfolds by itself when a man and a woman put the basic elements in correct alignment. With magnetic rods meeting at their opposite ends, the circular energy can flow.

This circle is more likely to happen spontaneously when a man and a woman are in love. If they are not in love, it will be a meeting of sex centers—one positive pole with one negative pole. There will be an exchange of energy, but it will be linear energy, not circular. This is the reason why sex without love is never very satisfying.

Femininity, arising through inner awareness, is magically magnetic. The inner focus, the joy of resting within herself, compels the male, who is equal and opposite in every way. A man will feel himself overwhelmingly and irresistibly drawn across a room to a certain woman. Suddenly there is a space, a vacuum, a receptacle into which his energy can flow effortlessly. In man a deep restfulness and satisfaction arises when his energy is received and absorbed and returned to him. Woman, in being loved, becomes love as the heart center grows more and more vibrant. Orgasmic states begin to arise when you relax into electromagnetic cooperation within and between female and male bodies.

The Seven Chakras

The positive and negative poles also fit into the esoteric system of the seven energy centers (chakras) that are present in the body. These are connected to five further energy centers that bridge us with universal consciousness, the energy of creation. The first energy center is located in the perineal/genital area of the body. The second, sometimes called the *hara,* is a few centimeters below the navel. The third is the solar plexus. The fourth is the heart. The fifth is in the throat. Sixth is the "third eye" between the two eyebrows. The seventh is at the top of the head and is called the crown chakra.

In the female body the first chakra is negative (vagina), the second positive, the third negative, the fourth positive (breasts), the fifth negative, the sixth positive, the seventh negative. The male body is opposite, starting with the first chakra as positive (penis), alternating upward with the fourth chakra as negative (heart).

The Healing Power of Magnetism

Magnets basically create order around them by aligning objects in their presence. You no doubt remember the earliest school science experiments demonstrating this. When iron filings are scattered on a sheet of a paper with a magnet lying underneath, the magnet demonstrates the field around it as the particles align themselves with the flow of magnetic energy between the positive and negative poles. When two magnets are placed apart under the paper with opposite poles facing each other, you can see the magnetic field in the circle of iron filings between the magnets themselves. In addition, the overall magnetic field surrounding the two magnets is infinitely greater than the field formed around a single magnet.

Plants and animals respond to a magnetic flow of energy through them that is induced by magnets. Today the use of magnets for their healing properties is becoming more and more respected.[2] They can be worn, for instance, as insoles, wrist bands, or kidney belts. Healing occurs because magnets provoke the magnetic flow of energy through the body. For example, photographs of unhealthy blood will initially show the individual cells in a random and chaotic arrangement. A second photo taken after a week of magnet therapy will show a semblance of alignment emerging between the cells of the body tissue. A week later again, the tissue will show an increasing order and formation developing in the cellular arrangement. The subject usually feels a relief in symptoms and an increase in well-being.

With all of this understanding of magnetic energies, the inner human magnet remains underdeveloped and unexplored. This is a sad state of affairs because the source of the orgasmic experience is precisely the same magnetic streaming between the female and male aspects within us. As these poles are gradually brought back into action and reestablished, energy organically flows between the positive and negative, bringing the body into a rare state of vibration. Realigning these magnetic poles in our bodies is a healing process in itself, and it starts with beginning to respect the feminine polarity within. Instead of playing out a male idea of how a woman is, our healing comes from being an actual woman: allowing ourselves to fall into the female element of receptivity and absorption—in other words, more being and less doing. With this *being* we discover what happens in the body when we focus on the vagina and the breasts. In conventional sex the vagina and breasts are sorely misused and this is affecting woman's orgasmic capacity. Right attention to the breasts and the vagina will be our focus in the next two chapters.

Tantric Inspiration

How to manage it [ecstasy]? Out of this question the whole science of Tantra was born. How to do it? It can be done. It cannot be done *with* the beloved outside—it cannot be done *without* the beloved outside, remember that too, because the first glimpse comes from the beloved outside. It is only a glimpse, but with it comes new vision that, deep down inside yourself, there are both the energies present—male and female.

Man is bisexual—every man, every woman. Half of you is male and half of you is female. If you are a woman, then the female part is on top and the male part is hidden behind, and vice versa. Once you have become aware of this, then a new work starts: your inner woman and inner man can have meeting and that meeting can remain absolute. There is no need to come back from the peak. But the first vision comes from the outer.

Hence Tantra uses the outer woman, the outer man, as part of inner work. Once you have become aware that you have a woman inside you or a man inside you, then the work takes on a totally new quality, it starts moving in a new dimension. Now the meeting has to happen inside; you have to allow your inner woman and man to meet.

OSHO, TRANSCRIBED TEACHINGS,
THE BOOK OF WISDOM

Awareness and Sensitivity Exercises
Partner Exercise to Awaken Polarity

This exercise can be done complete in itself or as a preparation for making love. Give yourselves at least thirty minutes.

Sit opposite one another on cushions situated a little distance apart so that you are without physical contact. (If sitting cross-legged on the floor is too uncomfortable, sit upright on straight-backed chairs facing one another.) Close your eyes. Inwardly tune in to your positive poles: woman tune to the breasts and man tune to the penis.

After a while imagine your breasts are radiating energy and light and warmth toward your man's chest and heart. Your partner should imagine himself receiving the love into his heart and at the same time channeling energy out through his penis, radiating warmth, light, and love. Imagine you receive all this energy and absorb it into your vagina. The imagination can be supported by radiating outward on the out breath (woman–breasts, man–penis) and absorbing on the in breath (woman–vagina, man–heart). You can breathe out together and in together.

After a while, begin to have eye contact with receptive, soft vision and continue circling the energy as before. After five to ten minutes, you (woman) can move across the space and sit with your legs wrapped around your man's waist while sitting in his lap. (This is called the yab yum position; cushions can be used to support the woman.) This brings genitals into closer proximity and the breasts and chest into correspondence. Again, keep working with your imagination, and this time you can experiment with synchronizing your breathing—as man breathes in through the heart, woman breathes out through the heart; as woman breathes in through the vagina, man breathes out through the penis. This practice will intensify the sensation of a circulating force between the bodies. If you do not feel this right away, after a time you will probably begin to feel it happening because energy follows imagination.

If yab yum is not comfortable to sustain for a period of time, you can move into standing position, or if yab yum is not at all possible the whole exercise can be done standing, to great effect. Standing allows for greater dance and fluidity of movement between bodies.

Spontaneously the wish to be penetrated may arise, and if your man is willing, continue with making love. Otherwise, when there is a sense of completion in the exchange, very, very slowly disconnect and move away from each other while maintaining eye contact. You can complete with a bow of the head with hands folded in a prayer gesture, or rest your foreheads together and then lie down on the bed or floor, side by side without contact (holding hands at most), and each rest within yourself for several minutes, keeping awareness on the inner streamings of the body (the magnetic rod).

Tantric Meditation
Peace Pervading the Armpits

Lie in a relaxed position as suggested at the end of chapter 1 for twenty minutes or more. Close your eyes, taking your awareness into your body. Start just between the two armpits, and with your total attention "pervade an area between the armpits into great peace."[3] Forget your whole body; remember the heart area between the two armpits and your chest and feel it filling with great peace. When the body is more relaxed, peace automatically happens in your heart; it becomes more silent and harmonious. Done frequently, this practice will establish peace within you and make you feel more independent, and love will be more about giving—you have so much peace you want to share it. You will be returning to a source in yourself that is always there.

5
The Breasts: Key to Orgasm

The breasts have the power to bring woman to the deepest of orgasmic experiences. The breasts are central to a woman's experience of sexual ecstasy, not merely an appendage for breast-feeding and without implication for the female energy system.

It is true that, for most of us, breasts are not directly associated with female orgasm, although certainly many women are aware of an internal hook-up to the vagina that is quite sensational. This connection between breasts and vagina happens via the magnetic rod (as explained in the previous chapter), the ultimate source of orgasmic states.

Orgasmic moments transpire when essential elements align themselves. Tantra is based on the science of the body and its energy centers, with their electromagnetic polarities. On the psychological level an individual requires a certain innocence. Heightened states are not accidental, although people may accidentally slip into a heightened state naturally perhaps once in a lifetime, without actually knowing how it happened. With information about the role of the breasts in orgasm, a woman has more command over her orgasmic experiences. She can consciously begin to create those experiences, rather than leaving it all to man's actions or to chance.

Energy Raised from a Positive Pole

The significance of the breasts in female orgasm is enormous in that, generally speaking, *energy can only be raised from a positive pole,* not a negative pole.[1] This means that energy is awakened or activated from the positive pole *before* it flows toward the negative. In the female body, sexual energy flows *from* the breasts *to* the vagina. When breasts are pulsating with aliveness, the spontaneous overflowing of energy results in a vibrational resonance in the vagina, the opposite pole. Only when the vagina is vibrating in this magnetic response is it truly available for the beautiful event of penetration; is it truly sensitive and perceptive. A woman will experience a genuine *yes,* a deep willingness to make love, a willingness not only to yield and give in but to participate fully as an equal and opposite—which changes everything, as if lifting sex to a higher octave.

The sexual route conventionally taken is very different because in it the vagina is regarded as the doorway and is approached directly (this will be discussed further in chapter 6). Indeed, while the vagina is the physical entry point, to energetically enter a woman the breasts must be given priority and consciously incorporated into the sexual exchange. Breasts are quite often ignored by women and men; certainly they are misunderstood in terms of their true role in accessing female sexual energy. If a man is into breasts, more often than not he uses them for *his* stimulation, to turn *himself* on, to fulfill some fantasy of his own, often treating the breasts very roughly in the process. The effect can even be to turn a woman off, causing her whole body energy to shrink into an unwillingness for sex. The naked truth is that regardless of the appearance of a woman's breasts or a man's personal interest in them, breasts represent the key to women's sexual fulfillment through orgasm.

Sadly, many women carry complexes about their breasts for any of a hundred and one reasons—the size, the shape, the hang, the fullness, the balance, the texture, plus all the variations possible in nipples. This lack of self-acceptance creates a tension and distances a woman from the delicate inner sensations present in her breasts. Emotional injuries, heartbreaks, and childhood wounds also can create energetic shields across the positive

pole. At first these tensions and repressed feelings can make it more difficult for a woman to feel into her breasts, until she learns to access the
power lying within them.

When a woman allows this magnetic phenomenon to come into play,
she begins to truly enjoy sex—sometimes for the first time. Not with the
feeling of having to fulfill a duty, submitting and enduring it, but with a
joyfulness that enables her to flower into a dancing sexual being. As the
breasts are brought more into the sexual forefront, orgasms will happen
more easily. Many different kinds of delightful orgasms will follow from
the breasts being lavishly included in lovemaking. Naturally, this involves
man—how he caresses and touches the breasts—but only to a certain
extent. At the deepest level it involves a woman's interest in herself as an
expression of the feminine.

You are encouraged to start feeling and sensing your breasts from
within. Do not be distracted by how they look from the outside, but
instead focus your attention on the breasts themselves. *It is best to keep
attention on both breasts at the same time.* Avoid long periods of focus on
one breast only. Spread your awareness over both of them: feel them, love
them, accept them as they are. Negative thoughts separate you from their
feminine qualities. Place your attention on the breasts, not with fierce
concentration, but more with ease and relaxation, with the sense of melting *into* the breasts, merging with them, becoming one with them.
Massage them, hold them, feel them from within at any time during the
day—as you set about working on the computer, cooking, gardening, or
whatever you happen to be doing. Whenever you remember, make an
effort to sense the breasts *from within.* And especially enter the breasts with
your awareness while making love. You will have to remind yourself of this
again and again, as our attention tends to stray easily to other things. The
breasts are the gateway for woman and need to be showered with all the
attention they can get—in and out of bed.

Even though most women do realize that the breasts are connected
with sexual pleasure, few really grasp how central and how intimately
linked their breasts are to full involvement in the sexual act and orgasm.
As mentioned earlier, fresh insight into the breasts puts a woman in a

better position to orchestrate events to her advantage, so as to let things flow in accordance with her feminine nature. A surprising number of women tell me that they always knew, intuitively, the truth about not forcing orgasm and about the role of the breasts in orgasm. Because of the pressures of conventional sex they had overridden their inner voices, not trusting themselves or their bodies. Some women have stood before me, eyes brimming with tears in the awesome realization that for twenty or thirty years they had been acting in direct opposition to their very essence. They feel so much time lost, opportunities missed, misunderstanding, and unhappiness as a consequence.

Fortunately, as far as the body is concerned, it is *never too late* to start changing our approach. The body welcomes all respect given to it, and in acknowledgment responds in beautiful and unexpected ways. The body is innately sensitive (our own insensitive and callous ways with it notwithstanding) and extremely responsive to *awareness.* Awareness means the sensing of the body from within; it means getting in there and feeling oneself on a cellular level.

Some women say they find it quite easy to sense the energies and sensations present in the heart area but not in the breasts, and they wonder if it is favorable to go directly to the heart. Even if the heart center is easily available, I nonetheless suggest that they tune in to and slowly awaken the life energy of the breasts. Ignoring the breasts and going directly to the heart may seem the easiest strategy, but it is a rejection of the essential feminine nature. Breasts access exquisitely delicate energies and surround a woman with the fragrance of femininity. Through the breasts the heart center is activated. In a sense a woman does not have to concern herself directly with the heart center. The heart opens as a by-product of the breasts becoming alive, and through this expansion of energy woman becomes increasingly loving, feminine, graceful, and elegant.

When you first begin to experience the breasts in a different way it is possible that some sadness or tears will surface. This is not at all unusual and is actually a good sign—a sign of your positive pole beginning to cleanse and free itself of earlier unexpressed feelings from hurts and heartbreaks that have accumulated energetically around the heart center. These tensions are released and the body purified automatically, through its intrinsic healing capacity, when a woman begins to amplify the positive energy present in her breasts. In this framework of cleansing, any tears and crying are to be welcomed, not shunned. Allowing them can bring profound healing of earlier unresolved issues. With each layer of tension that leaves the breasts and heart there will be a noticeable increase in the sensitivity and receptivity of the breasts. Some women carry a sensation that they describe as feeling like a metal plate of some kind across the heart. Energetically such a shield exists, but it is quick to melt when the environment is favorable. Past tensions can show up for release at any time—before, during, or after making love—so maintain an openness to yourself as much as possible.

The two nipples are the highlights of the positive pole, super alive and sensitive. Nipples have the ability to emit and radiate energy, making them similar to the head of the male penis. *Always bring both nipples into the focus of your attention* when feeling into the breasts as a whole. The nipple should be in the foreground of your awareness. Nipples are extraordinarily, deliciously sensitive and should be treated with love and respect.

Often nipples are twisted and turned roughly, like a couple of buttons. This can be very stimulating in effect, especially when a woman is younger. As women get older (and numerous women have reported this to me), they frequently find themselves rejecting almost all touching of the breasts, particularly of the nipples. Breasts and nipples that once were gloriously receptive and alive, that loved to be touched and played with, slowly become hypersensitive and overcharged, or deadened. A form of repulsion sets in because the rightful place of breasts (in the role of awakening female sexual energy) is not granted to them. In time a woman's instinctive reaction is to turn away from man's hands as they approach the vicinity of the breasts.

Touching the Breasts

Creating new experiences naturally involves the cooperation of the man to a certain extent, so encourage your man to touch your breasts in a way that feels good to you. Help him learn how to treat the breasts with love and awe. Some men are hesitant to touch the breasts because of earlier reactions and rejections, either by you or by a previous woman. This makes it really necessary to show him *exactly how* to touch your breasts in the way *you best* like your breasts to be touched, as suggested in the partner exercise at the end of the chapter. This is an intimate and beautiful step in taking responsibility for your own sexual expression. Show your man how to touch (or suck) your nipples and how to touch your breasts, separately and together. A man's two hands are not always available while making love. If only one of your man's hands is at your breast, touch the other breast yourself to give a feeling of balance.

Seek always that your man touch you in a way that *makes your body energy expand.* This sensation becomes the guideline for how to evaluate touch—look for an expansion of energy rather than excitement or stimulation. Avoid types of touch that create a contraction, withdrawal, or closing of your energy body. Light (and extremely featherlight), caressing touches have the effect of expanding and bringing sparkling sensations, while a heavy touch can reduce and deaden the pleasant sensations already present.

Touch your own breasts as often as possible while making love, any time it feels right or when you wish to deepen the connection to your inner experience. Touch your breasts simply and in the way that *you* most enjoy. This is the beauty of self-touch—you can do it however *you* like it, which brings a certain relaxation.

Cupping each breast lightly with your whole hand is a simple, loving way to touch the breasts. You can also cross your arms and cup each breast with the opposite hand (the right breast in the left hand and the left breast in the right hand). Keep your hands and fingers relaxed and open, shaping to the form of the breast. Give the breasts space; avoid squashing them too much. The palm of your hand automatically touches the nipples, which is a good thing because it will intensify the experience of the nipples. Soft caressing and stroking of the breasts is very nice, and especially erotic are the sides of the breasts as you lightly stroke upward from the armpit or side of the ribcage toward your nipples. Cupping and vibrating your breasts very gently from time to time also works wonders! Whenever you like, lightly stroke or squeeze the nipples just enough to produce fine sensations. A little saliva enhances the nipples' sensitivity. As you keep touching yourself in different suitable ways, you will feel the breast and heart awakening, filling up with energy and creating a pleasing response in the vagina.

There is another advantage to touching oneself that is completely unrelated to sensation. It can easily happen when another person touches us that we unconsciously and reflexively go on guard in fear of a touch that is uncaring or painful. Memories of these kinds of touch can come up. This fear, this tension, this contraction blocks the ability to deeply receive from the touching hand, to absorb the warmth and energy and love. With touching oneself there is no likelihood of this withdrawal happening.

Perhaps you feel a bit shy or self-conscious about touching your own breasts in front of your lover. But breasts have been the domain of the man until now, and it's time for a change. The effects are surely worth the risks. Gather courage and begin to express yourself in a different way. *Take risks each time you make love and you will be rewarded with love.* Every occasion you make love is an opportunity to experiment and explore, to check things out to see where your curiosity brings you. It really is best *not* to wait for *next time* to be adventurous. This postponement will continue as days all too quickly accumulate into years. If you wish to get out of the male-oriented sexual routine of today—and it is possible—you absolutely must take risks. Don't be overawed by man, by what he thinks or what he likes. Woman has been pleasing man in sex and moving away from her female expression for far too long. It is time for woman to take her place as the true counterpart in lovemaking that she is, and begin to please her body and cooperate with its inner mechanisms. Lucky is the man whose life will be enriched through her adventurous spirit.

Breasts and Excitement

A certain kind of touch or stimulation of the breasts by a man can produce a sudden surge of excitement or a desire to have a peak kind of orgasm. You might experience it as a real compulsion, an overwhelming urge that you simply *must* go with the desire and follow it through to the end. Touch or stimulation provoking this effect should be avoided or modified a little, perhaps offered more softly or with less intention. A relaxed, easy, caring touch will enable the deeper magnetic response to gather in woman and not flip her over into a state filled with desire for excitement and conventional orgasm.

Any hard squeezing, sucking, and stimulation of the nipples will often have this instant turn-on effect. But it can also have the entirely opposite effect—of turning a woman *off*, suddenly leaving her with no wish to go further. Which way she will react depends on the individual woman, her age, and how she has been handled by men in the past. Each unpleasant experience leaves a cellular imprint, a memory in the cells of the body, that creates a subtle barrier and layer of protection. (We will consider this again in chapter 6, in relation to the vagina.) Conscious melting of a man's hands into the breasts without squashing or squeezing them—not doing anything special other than sensing the breasts, feeling the energy of the breasts, loving them—works wonders. Avoid overstimulating the nipples, especially in the early stages of lovemaking or foreplay. *It is appropriate to touch and squeeze the nipples with more firmness when sexual arousal is complete and lovemaking well underway.* When the energy is flowing freely, the pressure to the nipples can cause delightful things to happen.

Direct and invincible evidence of how crucial the breasts are is that loving stimulation of the breasts encourages and increases lubrication in the vagina. Almost all women experience this. Through the magnetic link and overflow of energy, the lubrication glands in the vagina respond abundantly. In fact, there is a great deal more lubrication when the breasts are lovingly touched compared to when the vagina or clitoris is touched directly in foreplay prior to penetration.

Women who have had a breast removed for medical reasons report that the positive pole continues to be active *even in the absence of the physical breast.* The same filling up and spilling over into the vagina happens, as does the lubrication of the vagina. This remarkable feedback bears witness to the integrity of the body. The breast is more than just juicy flesh; it deeply embodies an energy dimension that remains active even in its physical absence.

A woman with one breast removed shares her experience: "When I touch my right breast in a delicate, quick, patting way, my vagina responds—it twitches and quivers and a wonderful wavelike, joyful current of sexual energy flows through my vagina, from the womb outward right to the vulva and clitoris. I can even feel the spot of my nipple and its connection to the vagina, although on the right side there is no physical breast anymore; there is only a thirty-centimeter scar.

"I am happy! It is so beautiful. With conscious loving touch and holding of the right breast 'in the air' as it were, it is fantastic. Sometimes I even feel the sensations more strongly and more vaginally than with the left breast. Interesting enough is that this most often occurs when sex is happening with heartfulness. With 'horny sex' I experience the touching of my scar as stimulating, often in the clitoris, but definitely much less than with the left breast. My partner is very sensitive; he can even feel the vibration of the nipple on the outside of the absent breast. I experience the energetic touch as a deep vaginal opening, and it creates a longing of the heart for deep touch.

"Since we discovered more about sexuality our sexual life has clearly moved in the direction of the heart and is creating a supportive, loving, divine atmosphere. One time after a deep union of hearts my lover shared, 'In the beginning it mattered to me. I was having thoughts about your having only one breast, particularly because I am attracted to big breasts. But now I feel everything is totally fine, as long as the heart is present and can be felt between us.' Sometimes my mind becomes doubtful, thinking: 'This isn't possible; this is just a scar! You're crazy, you're just imagining things!' And then I observe that in tandem with the negative thinking, the pleasing sensations are instantly gone. Then I feel into my body, into my vagina, and the moment I am able to accept my situation, and my lover touches *both* breasts a little more quickly, I again feel a strong twitching in my vagina. And there they are again: my two breasts! One time, lying naked in the sun after a deep penetration by my lover, I could distinctly feel my right breast when I touched it energetically, "in the air" so to speak. Because I am a skeptic, I immediately tried to just imagine being touched. I could feel something then too, but the sensation was much less than compared to the energetic touching by a conscious, loving hand.

"I received my diagnosis of breast cancer in 1993. My life had been ruled by fear, abuse, many years of drug use, a heavy and closed heart, and a certain longing to die. By means of awareness, with the help of countless workshops, meditations, and therapeutic groups, my life has transformed into conscious enjoyment, into a deep love of the universe, of life, with often a childlike joy and ease. My longing for real love, letting go, trust, flowing, inner peace, and connectedness has come true."

Deliberate Interference with the Breasts

It is extremely fashionable for women to have their natural breasts altered; in some countries it is considered normal to have artificial breasts, and a woman who has not had a breast enlargement is something of a rarity. As body piercing gains popularity around the world, some women choose to pierce their nipples, others their lips, and others their labia. And it seems that as the sexual confusion increases generation by generation, these types of enhancement and ornamentation are done at an increasingly young age.

In light of the crucial role of the breasts in female sexual energy circulation, cosmetic surgery to breasts raises certain issues. Fortunately, it is clear from the personal experience reported here that interventions do not ultimately destroy the energy intrinsic to breasts. It is also true that a woman's incentive and wish to be proud of her breasts is quite possibly a reflection of her intuition that her breasts play a dynamic and creative role in the sexual exchange, and therefore in her life. The urge to display her breasts to man naturally follows, and so the media and fashion world use exposed breasts in any way possible. One might say it's a good thing that men have greater opportunity to appreciate breasts through such displays. A woman's intention to display the positive, radiant pole is laudable—but sadly, her focus is misdirected. She is focused outward toward man, not inward toward herself. Breast enhancement surgery fixates a woman on the *outside* of her body, on her external appearance, not on how she feels internally. It then is not so easy to turn around, look within, and access the inner sensations of living breast tissue.

Some women have breast reductions because their breasts are so uncomfortably large that they become a physical and psychological burden to live with. In these circumstances, reducing the size can be considered a medical intervention and of psychological benefit. It can also be argued that increasing the size of the breasts puts a woman more at ease, gives her more confidence and trust in herself and her powers of attraction; in other words, that it benefits the woman herself. The added fullness of the breasts may result in attracting the male attention that a woman wants, but at a subtle level she might unconsciously begin to protect her breasts because they feel delicate. As a result she may be perhaps not so willing to let a man touch them. Men have shared with me that they can sense this, and that they will stay away from touching a woman's breasts in these situations. The breasts can feel uncomfortable; scars are sensitive, some never really healing properly. Artificial breasts have been known to explode during air flight! All these disturbances can easily affect the expansion of energy from the positive pole.

A woman might question whether encouraging a man to lust after her perfect breasts really serves her orgasmic potential in the long run. When a woman loves her own breasts and allows a man to love her breasts, they respond to the positive attention. Many women report an increase in breast size after they begin to make love according to female and male polarity—through bringing the breasts into their rightful magnetic alignment. Uncalled-for intervention of the breasts is a disturbance that interferes with the delicate magnetic system given to woman by nature.

A young and quite beautiful woman I met in a workshop told me she had enhanced her breasts two years earlier, saying, "You know, it was one of those things I just had to do, and after I did it I realized that I need not have done it." She had been thinking of reversing the operation, but after receiving the information on the importance of the positive pole, she decided that for the present she would finally accept her breasts as they are now and not interfere a second time. She was pleased, and relieved, to observe an overflow from her breasts to her vagina when she began making love using tantric principles.

Tantric Inspiration

This concentration at the breasts, melting into them, will give a new feeling to the female meditator—a new feeling about her own body, because from the center now she can feel the whole body vibrating. Just by loving the breasts of a woman she can be brought to a deep orgasm because the negative pole automatically will go on responding.

If you start from the breasts, meditating on the nipples, don't follow the route that you have read in books because that is meant for men. You simply don't follow any chart; allow the energy itself to move. It will happen this way; just a vague suggestion that first your breasts will become filled with energy, they will radiate energy, they will become hot, and then immediately your vagina will respond. And only after your vagina responds and vibrates, kundalini for you, for women, will start working. And the route will be different and the way the kundalini will arise will be different. In man it arises very actively, forcibly. That's why they have called it the serpent rising. Very forcibly, suddenly, with a jerk, the serpent unfolding. And it is felt on many points. Those points are called chakras. Wherever there is resistance the snake forces itself. It is just like the penis entering the vagina: the passage is similar for man. When the energy arises it is as if the penis inside is moving.

This will not be the feeling for a woman. The feeling will be quite the opposite. When woman feels that the penis has entered in the vagina— the melting sensation, the welcoming, the vagina giving way, vibrating very, very delicately, in a very receptive mood, loving, welcoming—the same will be the phenomenon inside. When the energy rises, it will be a receptive, passive rise, as if a passage is opening—not a serpent rising, but a door opening, and a passage opening, and something giving way. It will be passive and negative. With men something is entering, with women something is opening, not entering. Everything will be just the opposite. It must be so. It cannot be similar. The ultimate thing will be the same.

OSHO, TRANSCRIBED TEACHINGS,
THE BOOK OF SECRETS

Awareness and Sensitivity Preparation
Self-Massage of the Breasts

Massaging the breasts on a regular basis helps to reinforce the feelings of life force (also called *chi, energy,* or *prana*) present in the breasts. You will notice them becoming more sensitive and receptive. You will find it easier to get a feeling of them from the inside any time you put your awareness in them. Self-massage also helps you get to know your own breasts, to accept them, and to love them. Use body lotion or massage oil if you like. Breasts are ideally always massaged upward or in a circular motion, the left breast counterclockwise and the right breast clockwise. Lift the breast tissue upward as much as possible and include your chest and throat.

This practice is also a natural way of monitoring any changes in the breast tissue. If anything feels abnormal, is painful or itchy, is not associated with the onset of menstruation, and does not disappear after a short time, report it to a doctor immediately. It is not necessarily a cause for alarm, but have it checked as soon as you've detected it.

It is also beneficial to include with the breasts a deeper massage on the rib cage. Using your thumb or first two fingers braced together, make little circling movements that reach through your skin to the bone. Start with the breastbone (sternum), traveling up and down two or three times. In the center of the breastbone, on a line with the nipples of upright breasts, is the "love-spot"—an important energy point that lies over the thymus gland. Massaging here stimulates the immune system and is also a doorway to the heart. On each side of the breastbone is a series of little hollow spaces between the ribs, where the ribs join the sternum. These are called the intercostal spaces. Massage of these points encourages the growth of the breasts and also relaxes physical and emotional tensions. Massage the intercostal spaces using the fingertips in the circular way described above. It is also good to extend the massage to the ribs themselves, using a circling motion on the bone and between the bones; you can track the ribs with your fingers as they run behind the breasts and into the armpit area. You can also reach certain parts of the ribs by getting your four fingers under and behind the pectoralis muscle (the muscle that forms the front of the armpit and runs across the chest). You can use this massage sequence as complete in itself, as foreplay before making love, or followed by the tantric breast meditation below.

Partner-Exchange Exercise
Partner Exchange Massage for Breasts and Penis
It helps to show and teach each other how you like to be touched, communicating what opens and resonates in your body. Focus on touching with warmth and love; avoid the kind of touch that is intentionally stimulating and therefore has different effects. The aim is for the body energy to expand and flow first, not to arouse the body into excitement by touch. Put aside forty minutes or more for this exchange, depending on whether you wish to make love afterward, which is quite likely to happen.

Take several drops of unscented massage oil (such as almond or olive oil) in your hands and begin to touch and massage your own breasts with oil, showing your partner what pressure your breasts enjoy and what they do not respond well to. Show him how you prefer the nipples to be touched—or maybe not touched, perhaps just held by the palm of the hand. Share in this way for a few minutes, explaining as you go along, and then pour a few drops onto his hands so that he is able to continue massaging you in the way you most appreciate.

Lie back or sit up and absorb his caresses into your breasts for fifteen or twenty minutes. In general, the lighter the touch the greater the sensuality; featherlight works wonders. After completing this part, your man should do the same by showing you how to touch his penis and testicles, and then allowing you to take over the massage.

The orientation in this exchange is toward increasing feelings of aliveness, of awakening, but not directly toward any stages of full-blown excitement, where we get overwhelmed with desire. After a further fifteen to twenty minutes of the woman loving the penis with her hands, if it feels appropriate continue with a very slow penetration. All subsequent movements should happen in an unhurried, lazy manner.

Tantric Meditation
Meditating on the Breasts

Lie down alone in the ideal position for relaxation suggested in chapter 1, with about twenty minutes for yourself. Breast meditation can be done daily and will greatly support your breasts in coming to life and encourage the opening of your positive pole. If you have a lover, you can also use it as a part of foreplay or preparation for love, either on your own or with your partner lying in bed beside you.

If you wish, place a slightly cupped hand on each breast. Touching will enhance the feeling within the breasts, making it easier to bring awareness into them. If your elbows become uncomfortable at any time, change the position of your hands, placing them on the groin or lying with your arms straight at your sides. Close your eyes and take your awareness into your body, sensing your breasts and in particular your nipples. "Feel the fine qualities of creativity permeating your breasts and assuming delicate configurations."[2] Move into your breasts; let your breasts become your whole being. Melt into them, merge into them. The whole body can become secondary to the breasts; the body can fade into the background as you bring the breasts into the foreground. Your inner emphasis is on the breasts, totally relaxing in them, moving in them. Do this for twenty minutes and then simply rest for a few more minutes. True feminine creativity arises when the breasts become active.

6

The Vagina Is Secondary to the Breasts

The vagina plays a secondary role in a woman's orgasm—secondary to the breasts but not secondary to the clitoris (which is the subject of the next chapter). Breasts are the positive pole in the female body and the vagina is the negative pole. Energy from the breasts overflows and internally ignites the vagina, which creates the full *yes* for penetration by man. The breasts are a little detour away from the vagina for man, a trip through the female energy system before he approaches the physical port of entry. Instead of forced or quick penetration without enough knocking on the door, there is a waiting at the threshold for the deeper invitation to man, which awakens in woman through the breasts. When a woman's vagina vibrates in magnetic response to her breasts being loved, she instantly recognizes her moment of sexual readiness—she knows without any doubt that she is ready. There is an involuntary movement toward the man, a seemingly magnetic attraction to his body, a yearning for intimacy, for penetration, a deep longing to unite. This moment is not a mind decision or a submission to someone else's desires or wishes. It is instead a completely spontaneous, energetic happening: from the depths arises an utter *yes* to man. To man the difference is electrifying and immediately perceptible. This welcome, this wholehearted and full-bodied response, shifts sex into a higher dimension, a dimension in which it becomes an electromagnetic celebration that leaves you satiated and radiant with love.

Energy Flows from Male into Female

The intrinsic properties of the vagina are passive and receptive, welcoming, silky, serene, sensitive. The vagina is not an external organ like the penis; it is an inversion, a canal providing flow into the body, a delicate muscular recess. It is not designed to take direct action but to exert an influence on the penis through the quality of energy present in its tissues.

The physical correspondence of the penis fitting into the vagina is not accidental. The design is like this *because energy flows from male into female,* not the opposite way.* This is the direction of flow—from penis into vagina, from plus to minus. Through a balance in polarity a doorway opens; energy streams upward through our internal energy channels.

The penis is therefore to be appreciated as a conduit for vital energy as well as for semen. Likewise, the vagina is the receptacle for this force as well as for the semen necessary for reproduction. Woman as the feminine, receptive force has the capacity to draw the male energy upward through her vagina, as if raising it to a higher frequency. The vagina melts around the penis and drinks the energy radiating from it. When the penis and the vagina are united in penetration they form one complete unit, one dynamic force and one passive force, a live electromagnetic circuit.

However, women report that the vagina is rarely involved in their experiences of real sexual pleasure. The presence of the penis alone is seldom sufficient to create any kind of heightened experience. Very few

---

*In advanced stages of tantic lovemaking, in which a heightened balance has been achieved between male and female poles, energy can flow back and forth between the two poles in such a way that woman will alternate between active and passive phases of sexual expression, and man will be correspondingly passive and active.

women report a type of vaginal orgasm in which the vagina reaches an extraordinarily heightened state of sensitivity, in which the penis produces an experience of pleasure that is infinitely prolonged, utterly ecstatic. The vagina needs to be reincorporated in lovemaking, to take its rightful place in accessing pleasure and the flowering of orgasmic states. In a manner of speaking, until the moment of penetration man walks around as half a unit, half a circuit, and woman exists as the other half of the very same circuit. We must begin to ask ourselves in what way these two half circuits can meet so as to maximize the built-in energy circuit.

It is here, at the level of the genital interaction, where perhaps the greatest confusion in sex lies. How should the vagina best relate to the penis? How should they conduct themselves when they get together? What would *they* want for themselves if we did not force our personal expectations on them? These are questions we don't normally even think of asking because our sexual past has proved to us that the backward and forward movements of the penis in the vagina is what sex is all about. Without this rubbing interaction between them we think sex is not feasible, and so it is a stretch to imagine that other pleasures really do exist.

The truth is that the vagina, as passive pole, ought to be maintained wide and easy, available to receive the maximum impact of the male energy. When the vagina is physically and energetically open, man is finally able to flow *into and through* woman, following the direction of energy flow from positive to negative.

The Vaginal Consequences of Conventional Sex

With no choices available to us in sexual expression we stick to one style of sex, a style that has many unfortunate consequences. The greatest disadvantage for a woman is that the vaginal tissues are adversely affected, their receptive qualities gradually deadened. In the first place, a man usually penetrates a woman well before her sexual temperature is sufficiently high for her to invite him in. Man basically wants to enter as soon as he has an erection, and this forced entry makes the vagina reluctant and defensive rather than welcoming and willing.

Second, once man has entered, the repeated friction of the penis against the sensitive, silky vaginal walls has another negative effect: the vagina changes from a highly perceptive and receptive canal into a toughened, protected one. With time an increasing lack of sensitivity develops within the vaginal cavity itself. When the vagina toughens up this way, its magnetic perception of the entering male half circuit is drastically reduced. The receptive, absorbent tissues are instead literally covered over with thickened skin. The tensions held in the vagina, which can show up sometimes as sexual excitement, form an artificial screen of positive charge, almost male in character, that hinders a woman from absorbing male energy.

Third, the physical movements of the pelvis that go with the usual sex routine add to the increasing insensitivity within the vagina. Extremes of pelvic movement amount to a woman using her vagina in an active way rather than a passive way. Movement converts the vagina into an active, doing, outgoing organ. And the vaginal canal gets physically restricted and narrower, which disturbs the subtle, receptive energies of the vaginal environment. We use the penis and the vagina to have a nice rub together because we do not have the sense of how they communicate and exchange energy through their magnetic polarities. When the vagina becomes shy because of forced visits, hardened through friction, and tightened through movement, all the necessary passive complementariness to the male dynamic is obscured.

It's important to realize that simultaneous to this desensitizing of the vagina, the penis is *also* becoming less and less perceptive. With accumulating years the male organ becomes highly congested, tense and overcharged, excessively positive. In the same way that the vagina cannot absorb, the penis fails to function as a transmitter of pure positive male energy. This distortion of our given polarities is the root cause of our lack of deep, moving sexual experiences. The good news is that the polarity is not destroyed—it is hiding beneath this screen of tension. Overcoming the sexual habits and patterns responsible for this step away from polarity is the most direct route to reclaiming femininity (and masculinity) and regaining our inborn sensitivity.

Preserve the Vagina as a Sacred Place for the Penis

The first disconcerting observation a woman may have is that when there is no movement in sex, she cannot feel very much at all going on with the penis in the vagina. This is clear evidence that her vaginal walls have toughened up through excessive stimulation; through aggressive, hard thrusting of sex; and also through fingers and synthetic objects being inserted into the vagina. A woman is encouraged to respect and preserve her vaginal sensitivity and to take special care about what enters the vagina and how. It is best to consider the vagina as a sacred place for the penis. Too many uncaring visits and invasions lead to loss of vaginal sensitivity, and from there, to reduced capacity to perceive vaginal pleasure and delight.

In the short term, most forms of direct stimulation inside the vagina may increase pleasure; but in the long term, more and more stimulation will be required to produce the same effect. Increasing numbness sets in as the body gradually forms a protective layer and becomes less and less sensitive to the stimulation. With objects and fingers there exists no real energetic correspondence, as there is with the penis during penetration. Objects can produce an effect through stimulation and resulting excitement, but they cannot possibly substitute for the profound effect of the living penis. A woman can resensitize her vagina through changing her style of lovemaking and learning to trust the power of receptivity.

Accessing Deeper Reaches of the Vagina, the Female Epicenter

It will interest women to know that the most meaningful part of the vagina is not the tighter entrance area, with its rings of muscle (which men like to focus on for stimulation), but the higher parts of the vagina, especially around the mouth of the uterus. It is here that the feminine pole is most negative and most receptive. This is where a woman is more likely to experience quite heavenly sensations and access altered states of consciousness. A woman will experience this phenomenon even if she has had her physical uterus and cervix removed. But this upper part of the vagina is usually not touched by the penis because the vagina is restricted and tense, in part to protect and guard against fast deep penetration. Most women, whether they are conscious of it or not, hold the upper part of the vagina tightly closed because it is *extremely* painful when the penis aggressively hits up against the cervix.

To allow a man to reach this most sacred focal point in woman—a place that can be thought of as the garden of love—she must keep the vagina relaxed. Essential for this is the prerequisite of a loving penis and, initially, an exaggeratedly slow penetration of the vaginal canal, millimeter by millimeter. One penetration to the very depths of the vagina can easily take several prolonged minutes, and even then perhaps the lovers will remain still for some minutes more before the need for further movement arises.

This style of deep penetration will bring the epicenter of the female pole, the area around the cervix, to correspond directly with the head of the penis, which is like a highly sensitive magnet. If the penis is unable to reach as high as the cervical area, women have reported that the cervix itself draws closer to the head of the penis. Between the negative cervix and the radiant positive penis head, a powerful interaction on an electromagnetic level occurs, with a catalytic discharge of the accumulated tensions that are lodged in the tissues causing insensitivity. The penis will have this effect in the vagina as a whole, and particularly in this upper region.

Healing Sexual Traumas with Deep Penetration

Many women carry forward into their lives the devastating emotional pains and tensions resulting from sexual abuse they suffered as young girls. Courageously they piece themselves together again to enter the sexual domain, sometimes as deeply wounded beings. Some fortunate women are able to get therapy to process the past, to work the feelings out of their energy system. While this is certainly helpful, there still remains a residue of the memory stored on a cellular level in the body, particularly in the vagina, the lower belly, and the ovaries. These disturbing memories may on occasion unconsciously get triggered, resulting in recurring emotional outbreaks and unhappiness as the woman reexperiences the negative vibrations of her past, still active inside her. (See chapter 10 for a more detailed discussion of emotions.)

All the old memories and feelings, stored as tensions, can be discharged by the penis—the very organ that did damage in the first place. Unconsciousness caused the damage; consciousness can heal it. Lack of love was the cause; love can heal it. The penis is able to gradually break up and discharge tensions and return vaginal tissues back to sensitivity and aliveness. In fact, most women will notice that the vagina has many painful places that only become discernible and evident when the vagina is more relaxed, having given up its guard, and when the penis is slow and loving. Pain almost always reflects tension, or it reflects a memory or an inner holding of some kind. The releasing of old tensions enacts a profound healing for the female psyche. (And the penis experiences the same kind of healing through this process.) The partner exercise at the end of this chapter provides practical details on deep penetration.

A woman shares her experience: "When we did the deep penetration I had a big energy release at my womb. It was very painful but at the same time it felt very good; it was almost unbearable. I understand now about how energy is stuck inside. I felt lighter afterward and I can feel my womb pulsing. But today I was even more aware of the tension. It is as if I'm noticing this tension for the first time, and the more I feel the release, the more aware I am of the tension."

A woman shares her experience: "About the deep penetration around the cervix—at first I felt beautiful sensations and joy and I had the image of having a very small gold treasure box in there. But that was very short-lived. After, it became an unbearable physical sensation right at the cervix. We had to stop many times because I could not take it, and all the time I was having an electrical discharge all over the body. It became more unbearable when we made love later that night. I had great discomfort, I was tense everywhere. Then I started to have the feeling of being at the doctor and I connected with the actual fear of physical pain right at the cervix. I remembered gynecological visits, where they touch there to take samples for tests, and the painful insertion of an IUD. As I talked to my lover about it the pain calmed down. In the morning I experienced total relaxation, silence, presence, and stillness as we made love."

A man (partner of the previous woman) shares his experience: "The love-making was very powerful in that a lot came up for my partner. It would be so intense for her that I had to come out several times. Finally something released and it was beautiful to feel her vagina relax and suddenly I started crying."

A woman shares her experience: "Today there was much pain released during the penetration, in my vagina and my heart. All the rapes came back. I had a big emotional outburst and found it difficult to accept that nevertheless it happened—and my vagina is feeling more alive and still very painful—so is my heart. For me right now it is an emotional phase. Cramps and pains, release in the vagina, vivid memories of different abuse stories, abortions, sterilization. Often tears come up and a deep mistrust and for the first time I see how the sexual abuse has wounded me, made me vulnerable, and much is opening up in my heart. I see the tendency in myself to trash that vulnerability with jokes and power games."

A woman shares her experience: "When I open, there is a flower in my vagina, deep inside, like at the cervix or thereabouts. I can speak from there. It is a welcoming. It is like another heart in my body. I have experienced this before but I never valued it."

A woman shares her experience: "Whenever the movements get too much for me, I say 'stop,' and my partner waits for a while and later begins moving again. We have found a form that is feeding our basic hunger, caring for our tissues' needs for exchange instead of friction, and we have become much more sensitive. When we go for friction sex every once in a while just to see what it's like, we both get so sore and itchy we have to wait a week before we are back to normal. All we need for our physical healing is simply putting the penis in the vagina! Speaking of which: the medicine

I had bought before our first workshop to heal my heavy fungus has been sitting in the refrigerator unused ever since. My vagina has never had fungus again!"

Healing is usually a process that happens in layers, sometimes gradually and sometimes more quickly. Do not expect immediate results or even instant ecstasy. Healing depends a great deal on how willing a woman is to relax into her nature and to release the past that she is carrying. When old feelings arise it is not essential to understand the source of trauma; if you do, great, but you need not search around for the reason why your tears are falling—simply dive into the feeling and express it. Otherwise you can get lost in thought and lose contact with the feelings welling inside. Women also carry pain on a collective level, for all of womankind and the tragedies of humanity.

Following a period of cleansing of old memories and pains, the polarity will be fully restored. Women will feel an ecstasy generated by the luminous, beaming penis head corresponding in its rightful way with the epicenter of the passive, absorbent vagina. In these moments a woman can also feel a vibration in the opposite end of the magnetic rod: in the heart and breasts. And many women report the experience that as the energy moves upward to reinforce the opening in the breasts, it is as if the penis actually penetrates the heart, the female positive pole. It becomes a full-bodied experience, radiating through arms, legs, and head—at times the sensation extends beyond the body, giving rise to a bodiless, floating sensation. The experience of penetration is not limited to sensations localized in the vagina. The vagina is the physical entry point of the female energy system, and as such the vagina is only part of the total experience.

The Breasts Impulse the Vagina and Expand Energy

When first "in" love, women report that they more easily have experiences of orgasm. This is true because the heart is naturally open, chest and breasts alive and vibrating in love energy. The vagina, at the other end of the magnetic rod, automatically begins resonating and answering.

As years pass lovers can lose their initial sensitivity and aliveness to themselves and to each other. Slowly, sex becomes more routine; each starts to take the other for granted and forgets to appreciate his or her partner's good qualities. This process is often accompanied by a diminishment of energy vibrating in the heart center. Sometimes this corresponds with the common experience of the "honeymoon being over," where suddenly something radiant but invisible evaporates. The sensation of being *in love* with a man becomes one of loving *him*. This in itself is fine, but life can become full of habits that distance us from the heart center and from our partner. For a woman, this distance can also affect her orgasmic capacity.

Fortunately, the converse is also true. When a woman approaches the sexual act with her breasts, in their organic sequence, the female positive pole vibrates, generating orgasmic states. *Being* in love becomes a daily reality.

To summarize, there is a circular movement in the female energy system that flows down first and then upward. Following polarity, the sexual energy awakens initially in the breasts and then overflows to the vagina before turning upward again to return to the heart. Any intensification of touch or awareness at the breasts at any time will create further overflow and intensification of experience, and will even enhance male erection. (See chapter 8 for woman's part in erection.) Sex that does not harness these body polarities becomes a linear experience leading to frustration and unhappiness, because the innate ecstatic potential of the meeting is completely forgone.

Tantric Inspiration

So just relax into each other and forget about the mind. Enjoy the very presence of the other, the meeting, and get lost in it. Don't try to make anything out of it; there is nothing to make. Then one day there will be a valley orgasm, there will be no peak. There will be only relaxation, but that has its own peak because it has depth. Some day the body will trigger itself into a peak orgasm but that will also be coming; you will just be there.

Sometimes there will be a valley, sometimes there will be a peak . . . and that is a rhythm. You cannot have a peak every day. If you have only peaks, then the peak will not be very big. You have to earn the peak by going into the valley. So it is half and half. Sometimes it will be a valley orgasm. Then get lost in the darkness of the valley, the coolness and the peace. That is how you earn a peak. One day the energies are ready: they themselves are going towards the peak. Not that you are taking them. How can you? Who are you and how can you manage to? By being in the valley the energy accumulates; the peak is born out of the valley. Then there is great orgasm; your whole being is suffused with a joy.

OSHO, TRANSCRIBED TEACHINGS,
THE OPEN SECRET

Awareness and Sensitivity Exercise
Building Consciousness in the Vagina

While standing equally balanced on two feet, relax and contract the pelvic floor to build awareness in the vaginal cavity. The pelvic floor refers to all the muscles surrounding the vagina and anus. These stretch in one direction between the coccyx to the pubic bone and crosswise between the two sitz bones. They form a web of muscles with the perineum in the center, situated between the anus and the vagina, as the focal point.

Slowly pull up and slowly relax, with your attention at this focal point of the perineum. You can also highlight the vaginal muscles at the front or the anal muscles at the rear. While doing so it is important to also relax the belly muscles, as many women unconsciously tighten the abdominals to give an impression of a flatter belly. A relaxed belly, one that protrudes, is of great advantage in that it maintains the balancing integrity of the arch in the lumbar spine. Allow the stretch in the lumbar area to come through the relaxation of the abdominal muscles and not through simply sticking out the buttocks, which is a form of tension. Search for this balance within yourself, and then consciously contract the muscles of the vagina for about 60 seconds of slow, rhythmic contractions.

Slow means *slow,* and you are likely to feel this as quite an effort. In time you can increase the number of contractions. When finished, immediately lie down with eyes closed and rest for five to fifteen minutes. While resting you can also get in tune with the magnetic rod running between your vagina and breasts, and relish any spreading of energy and warmth that may follow.

At any time during the day, make it a practice to bring awareness to the area around the vagina (and the belly) and relax it, wherever you are and in whatever you are doing. Tighten, relax, tighten, relax—no one can see, and it feels really good. With your awareness begin to focus inside the vagina to awaken the life already present in the tissues. You will notice again and again that the vagina is tightened (through unconscious fears and tensions), so simply keep relaxing whenever you remember to. When the channel upward is clear and open, any contractions are likely to result in ecstatic sensations pulsating upward to the top of the spine.

Partner Exchange Exercise
Deep Penetration and Healing the Vagina (and Penis)

You and your lover should develop deep penetration as a style of lovemaking, with your man focusing deep in the vagina whenever possible. The way to set about this is to ask your man, when he has an erection, to enter your vagina extremely slowly and to go as far in as he is able. Then hold still for a while, as described earlier in this chapter. Before your man penetrates you, open your labia (the vaginal lips) and hold your vagina open while he penetrates. Doing this will make the penetration smoother and more powerful.

In addition, it is an excellent idea to reach between your legs from time to time during lovemaking and open your outer labia. It really enhances the feeling of the penetration because of the increased correspondence—it is like a deepening kiss between penis and vagina. Simply reach your arms between your legs (your man may have to pull his body away a tiny bit, but without losing penetration), lay each hand alongside the vulval area, and with the fingers pull the labia apart, clearing the way as it were, pulling open the folds of tissue at the entrance of the vagina (inner labia) as well as extricating any pubic hairs that may have strayed there. You can keep your hands in this opening position for a while before withdrawing them from your pelvic area. When you have withdrawn your hands, your man can deepen his penetration by a few centimeters (which is worth more than it may sound). This procedure may seem like a bit of a disturbance, as your man has to back off for a few moments, but the increased sensations of pleasure in depth are clearly worthwhile.

With extremely slow penetration any painful places are likely to become apparent as the penis moves, or even lies still, in the vagina. Remember, pain anywhere is usually an indicator of some inner holding, and pain can be present at any point of the vagina, even right at the entrance. We must seek out these painful points with intention, with the penis, and bring the area into correspondence with the magnetic penis head. As mentioned already, the penis will still have an impact even if penetration is not to the full depth of the vagina.

Ask your partner to hold still when the head of his penis is touching any place that feels painful. Travel internally with your awareness to the area and feel into it from the inside. It is essential for the penis to have "porous" contact with your vagina, which means the head must not push with force into any tender area. Rather, once you have identified the discomfort—the point where you tell your partner to hold still—he should draw his penis back about a millimeter or two, a hairbreadth. This minuscule amount of space allows for an interchange of energies; otherwise the pressure of the penis will further compact tensions instead of loosening them.

You can contact your partner's eyes with soft vision or you can close your eyes, whatever feels appropriate at any given moment. As you rest in yourself, just see what you feel and allow whatever wants to happen, be it feelings of sadness that come up, any shivering or shaking—a gale of laughter may even suddenly erupt out of you. The deep penetration may only last a few minutes; sometimes the penis will relax down after it has done this work, and if you both remain relaxed and easy and allow it to lie in the vagina, resting, it might surprise you by rising up again into erection.

Possible Positions for Deep Penetration

A variety of positions are suitable for deep penetration. You can try them all. Each position allows the penis to engage with the vagina from a variety of different angles, giving the opportunity to explore every corner of the vagina. It is most useful for a woman to place a folded pillow or a small square cushion under her pelvis (as shown in figures 6.1 and 6.2) so as to raise the pelvis and increase the depth and angle of penetration.

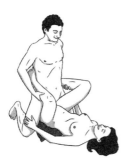

Fig. 6.1. Middle position, man kneeling (with pillow to raise woman's pelvis)

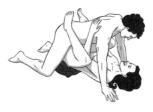

Fig. 6.2. Middle position, man on hands and knees (with pillow to raise woman's pelvis)

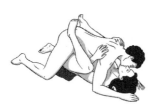

Fig. 6.3. Middle position, man lying forward, half kneeling (with pillow to raise woman's pelvis)

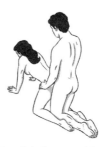

Fig. 6.4. Rear position

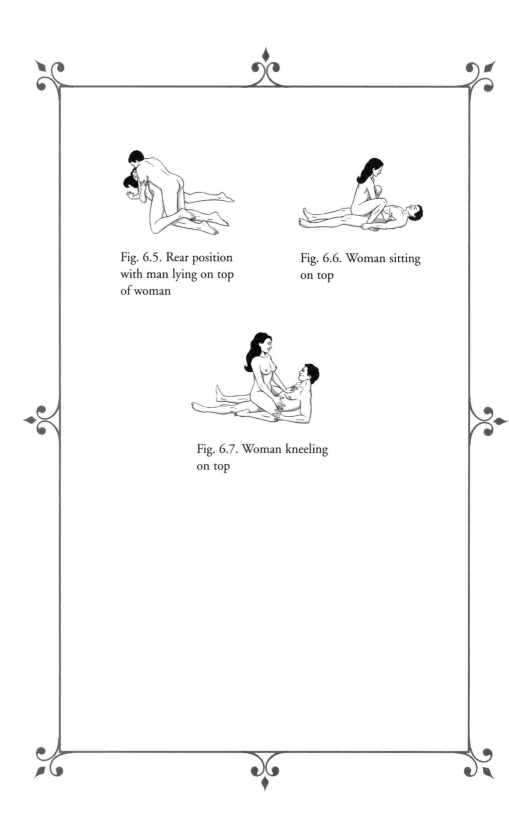

Fig. 6.5. Rear position
with man lying on top
of woman

Fig. 6.6. Woman sitting
on top

Fig. 6.7. Woman kneeling
on top

7

The Clitoris and Excitement

The clitoris has a beautiful place in the sexual exchange, but even with an incredible fifteen thousand nerve fibers that penetrate the pelvis and connect with the clitoris, it is not the center of female sexuality (as believed by most women today). The clitoris does not even rank a good second place; the breasts and the vagina are the true source of the orgasmic state. For many years now, we have placed undue emphasis upon the clitoris for female orgasm because we lacked wisdom and insight into the receptive aspect of the vagina.

Today more than 70 percent of women report that the vagina has little to do with their experience of orgasm and pleasure; instead, they rely on the sensations of the clitoris. This reality reveals the fact that male penetration is not very significant to most women, as far as their sexual satisfaction is concerned. It also implies that man has lost his ability to communicate meaningfully to woman through his penis. Instead of bringing her to heightened states, penetration usually leaves a woman high and dry, with no orgasmic experience at all. In the face of this situation, both men and women have resorted to directly stimulating the clitoris with the intention of producing a peak type of orgasm for the woman. The goal-oriented pressure and tension needed to "achieve" an orgasm (especially when the woman feels pressured to climax to please the man) can make it hard to climax at all or to do so in a satisfying manner. When we understand more about female sexuality, we can see that the clitoris acts as a great diversion for a woman. In seeking orgasm via the clitoris she is distanced from the feminine, receptive qualities of her vagina in relation to the penis. As a consequence, fulfilling sexual experiences become more and more elusive. The clitoris can certainly contribute intensely pleasurable experiences, but it is the vagina, which actually embraces the penis, that leads most directly to orgasmic states. To access these finer levels of sensitivity a woman needs to be willing to steer away from the clitoris and develop an interest in the vagina, the deep receptacle of her femininity.

Excitation Versus Excitement

It is essential to understand that direct stimulation of the clitoris produces sexual excitement, which is a form of tension. Tension causes contraction and inhibits energy from spreading, so it is not basic to the expansive orgasmic design. Perhaps differentiating between *excitation* and *excitement* will be helpful here. Excitation is a state of aliveness, of refined vibration, tingling, and inner delight. If such pleasing sensations are played upon or intensified through continued touch or stimulation, excitation can quite easily change character and shift into excitement coupled by an overwhelming urge for orgasm. Excitation is beautiful, wide, of the here and now, without direction—the pleasure is enough unto itself. Excitement is narrower; it has a direction and it rouses a compulsion to take the sensations to some overwhelming conclusion.

A woman is advised to stay with excitation as much as possible and to avoid excitement, especially during penetration. Woman's excitement has a peculiar effect on a man, with dire consequences—intensity of sexual excitement in a woman encourages early ejaculation in a man. Premature ejaculation is fostered when women get too excited either before or during the sexual act. If a woman always wants or needs a great deal of stimulation during sex, her partner is more likely to have a premature ejaculation problem. When a man attempts to arouse his woman through a lot of stimulation, he is ensuring that he will ejaculate soon. Some men ejaculate immediately before the much-dreamed-of penetration, totally overcome with excitement and anticipation. Others ejaculate within a few minutes. As we well know, loss of erection usually follows ejaculation, and man is disabled from staying inside woman for long enough to make any impact on her. (As to his experience, with this quick ejaculation man does not deeply sense that he has made love and so he begins longing for sex again, fantasizing about it, dreaming of the moment when he will penetrate again. As mentioned earlier, the mere discharge of semen does not grant a man the satisfaction that comes with deeper orgasmic states.)

Thus, a man is seldom inside of a woman long enough for either of them to experience the pure channeling of energy into the woman, and the glory of this. When the sexual energy is able to move in a circular way according to polarity, the penis is functioning finally as a conduit for male energy. However, because of his premature ejaculation, the man is unable to remain present in the vagina; this has made his woman dependent on her clitoris, and thereby on excitement, for sexual satisfaction.

If both parties to the sexual act remain relatively "unexcited," they can delay ejaculation for a long time and prolong the lovemaking. Ejaculation becomes a choice, not a necessity. To reduce the incidence of ejaculation *prior* to penetration, a woman should cool down during foreplay to ensure that her man stays relatively unexcited—that is, if she wants him to enter her. By reducing excitement she naturally makes her man more potent, putting him in more of a position to satisfy her.

The same principle of keeping it cool applies during penetration: keep the excitement level down so that man can continue to avoid ejaculation. When the excitement level and tension in the vagina get too high, a man will ejaculate, especially when the woman moves her pelvis in an active way in order to engage and stimulate the clitoris. The excitement of this is instantly communicated to the penis. Any sudden, urgent rushes of excitement should be avoided because these will virtually "pull" an ejaculation out of a man. Unless a man has authority, unless he is relaxed and in control of himself, he almost has no choice but to ejaculate. Men report in particular an uncontrollable discharge when a woman shifts gears and tries to intensify excitement so she can pull off an orgasm. One man described how he experienced this pulling sensation as a kind of dark substance entering and overwhelming him. Men themselves are amazed at how quickly an ejaculation can happen in the face of a woman's increasing excitement. Of course, if a man loses his erection, it hardly matters to the 70 percent of women who in any event rely on the clitoris; but this conventional approach limits female experience because it is removed from the penis and vagina—the organs of love themselves.

The Inclusive, Polarized Vagina

The vagina is an electromagnetic cavity, and *included* in it, not separate from it, is the clitoris. One pole ("positive") is found at the clitoris and the other pole ("negative") is found in the deepest part of the vagina, around the mouth of the uterus (cervix) and upper regions, as explained in chapter 6. An electromagnetic connection exists between these two poles, which runs through the so-called G-spot. (The G-spot is named after the gynecologist Ernst Grafenberg, 1881–1957, who was the first to offer a theory concerning this area.)

The G-spot is a highly erogenous cushion of tissue located just a few inches inside the vagina on the front wall, almost up behind the pubic bone. This is where the vagina wraps around the urethra (the tube that carries urine from the bladder). The area is connected to the sphincter muscles of the bladder, which may be one reason for its sensitivity. Added sensitivity can be attributed to the fact that the area forms the back end of the clitoris, which has nerve roots that run very deep.[1]

Recent research has established that the tissues of the G-spot contain an enzyme also found in the male prostate gland, suggesting that the urethral sponge may be the female version of this gland, which is also rather sensitive to pressure and touch in men. The existence of these tissues in this place may also explain the fluid secretions many women experience during or after G-spot stimulation. Sometimes called female ejaculation, copious sexual juices can be released from the G-spot. For some women, ejaculation happens in heightened sexual states; for other women, ejaculation is not accompanied by any special sensations.

There can be no question that every woman possesses a G-spot; what differs is whether or not she feels it. Each woman carries her personal sexual history, made up of individual physical and psychological factors that can interfere with her sensitivity. However, by now we know that the penis has the capacity to heal the vagina of past aggressions. This means in reality that, in time, any woman ultimately has the capacity to experience the joy of the G-spot. While this is true, it is rather hidden away inside the vagina—though most women can feel it if they probe gently into the vagina with a forefinger and explore behind the pubic bone/bladder area. During lovemaking the area can sometimes get engorged, making it easier to feel. In any case, the G-spot should not be made a separate focus of attention and thus interrupt the awareness of a woman from the *whole of the vagina*. All these mysterious parts *together* make up the incredible wonders of the female genitalia.[2]

And so it follows that the G-spot, like the clitoris and like the vagina itself, should be approached in a passive, easy manner, not sought after or hunted. Perhaps in certain angles of penetration the G-spot or the clitoris may come into play. A little further on we will consider how women can make use of clitoral possibilities. However, neither the clitoris nor the G-spot is the real source of orgasmic ecstasy for women.

Integrating the Clitoris without Disturbing the Vagina

We need to reevaluate the clitoris and find its place in deep, moving orgasm. We also need to appreciate the vagina and give value to the event of penetration—the conjoining of male and female poles—which will lead to higher experiences. The real art for women lies in integrating the clitoris without distracting from the vagina. To do this it is usually best to avoid stimulating the clitoris before penetration. As mentioned, excitement builds tension in the vagina. The vaginal environment physically contracts—

some women report a slight, dull ache—while turning slightly positive and unreceptive, which inhibits the potential electromagnetic streaming from the penis into the vagina.

I frequently ask women in my workshops if they notice whether the vagina is less sensitive or more sensitive to the penetrating penis after a bit of clitoral stimulation during foreplay. The overwhelming majority of women raise their hands to say that in fact they notice the vagina is *less* sensitive after the clitoris has been played with. They perceive the sensation and pleasure of penetration as tremendously heightened when the vagina is in a more innocent and passive state, undisturbed by any previous genital touching. (Remember, with tantric sex the vagina is already streaming with receptive energy from loving focus on the breasts.) This clearly demonstrates that stimulation of the clitoris creates tensions that make the penetration much less sensational. The stimulated clitoris seems to disturb the composure of the vagina, creating a restlessness, a wanting, a kind of hunger for orgasm that dramatically reduces the significance and intensity experienced in penetration itself. And once the penis is inside, the excited woman's tendency is to want to go for the orgasm (again by way of the clitoris) rather than to stay with the actual reality of the penis in the vagina.

If you choose to engage the clitoris during sex, it is much better to do so much further down the road—certainly well after penetration, perhaps even after an hour or two of making love. This time gives your body a chance to open fully via the energy channel between breasts and the vagina. Then, if the clitoris is approached in a relaxed, easy, passive way—as an extension of the vagina itself—it can deepen vaginal awareness, greatly intensifying sensitivity, and adding to orgasmic states.

The clitoris can therefore be used in two opposing ways: The first is as a direct doing, an active stimulation—with the outcome of making woman a bit pushy and easily orgasm-oriented, which reduces her awareness in the vagina. Or the clitoris can be used in a non-doing, more passive, softer way, which makes a woman more receptive and open and increases awareness in the vagina. One way leads to discharge, the other way leads further into her ecstasy and femininity.

So in general it is advisable to leave the clitoris unstimulated to a certain extent. The temptations of the clitoris are enormous because it does feel delicious, but in truth the clitoris should serve as a bit of fun now and then, not as the basis of your orgasm or sexual experience. On occasion the clitoris will unexpectedly, happily chime in with everything else and further heighten your experience. But without an orgasmic base—the vibration of the magnetic rod between the breasts and vagina—the clitoral orgasm is not usually deeply moving, and can leave women in an emotional state.

The Clitoris as Bridge to the Vagina

Certainly peak orgasms do feel good in themselves; but they beckon us away from the orgasmic state—the relaxed expansion (of the same energy) that lies at the other end of the spectrum. However, some women report that through stimulating the clitoris and having a quick peak orgasm, they can relax more into their orgasmic nature. The quick release skims off tensions present in the system, and this can have a relaxing effect on a woman. And relaxation is basic to orgasm. When relaxed, a woman will suddenly feel more sensual, feminine, and receptive, with the vagina more available. So a woman *can* use the clitoris as a bridge to the vagina, but if she peaks in this way during penetration she gets there at some risk to herself. As we know, man easily ejaculates with the final onrushes of female excitement, thus ending the approach to her deeper orgasmic state.

Some women also say that a bit of clitoral stimulation can raise their temperature to a full *yes* to penetration. Some women, in experimenting, say it is a relief to turn away from the imperative to go all the way for a peak orgasm with the clitoris; instead, at some point it feels right to say, "That's enough, I want you *in* me now," and then to relax into penetration without effort.

Many women prefer oral stimulation of the clitoris to other types of clitoral stimulation because it's wet, it can be sensuous and silky, and there's no irritation from rough, calloused fingers. Even oral stimulation is not appreciated so much when it gets hard and fast and rhythmic—it builds too much tension, too much pressure to climax.

Oral (or any) stimulation of the clitoris requires a new attitude: it should be like a short visit just to say a loving hello and then to move on. Oral sex can be used in support of awakening the energy but not to produce a full-blown orgasm; it can be used in support of remaining in excitation states without getting overexcited.

As we know, many women don't even expect to reach orgasm during actual intercourse, with the penis in the vagina. Their peak results from some form of direct oral and/or manual stimulation of the clitoris, which is in fact most easily achieved without penetration. Or it comes from pelvic rocking to stimulate the clitoris during intercourse. (A woman might think, "Of course he's going to come before I do once he gets in there. That doesn't mean I need to give up peak orgasms. It just means I need to have a quick orgasm before he goes in, or manage one after he's come.") On top of this, clitoral stimulation is generally assumed to be essential to female orgasm.

But here is new information: One of the biggest differences between conventional sex and tantric sex is that, in the latter, women *can* experience orgasmic states with the penis in the vagina. In fact, penetration is a necessary part of how the polarities work together to bring us into the orgasmic state. Leaking the sexual energy through momentary experiences, pleasing though they may be, is ultimately not enriching or uplifting and neither is it empowering for a woman.

If a woman is curious about her clitoris and about exploring it from a completely different angle, it will be interesting to know that tantra recognizes the existence of a subtle nerve that connects the clitoris to the little hollow above the upper lip.[3] Gaining control over this secret nerve route can enhance the pleasures of lovemaking for woman and man. (See the awareness exercise at the end of the chapter.) During lovemaking this subtle channel can be activated through visualization. Then, a man can greatly enhance this activation by kissing the upper lip of his woman, gently sucking and tugging on it, thereby stimulating one end of the channel. At the same time the woman can, if she wishes, take the lower lip of her man into her mouth and do the same.

Identifying Desire and Separating from Urges

As you make love and monitor your excitement in an attempt to keep the climate cool, it is important to identify the precise point where the tide changes for you—where you suddenly feel an urgency for orgasm. This point is significant because here something creative can be done, if you are interested in transforming conventional sexual patterns. If a desire arises within you, tantra does not tell you to fight it. It is futile to fight with desire, but that doesn't mean that you become its victim or that you indulge in it. Instead tantra gives you a very subtle technique.

"When a desire arises, just at the beginning, just at the first glimpse, the first flicker of desire arising, be alert. Bring your total awareness, the entirety of your being to look at the arising desire."[4] Don't do anything, just face the desire squarely, in full consciousness, and relax back into yourself. Nothing else is needed. The energy falls back inside you, wells up, and expands powerfully through the body, lifting you to another level of experience and sensitivity. When desire disappears without a fight, it leaves you powerful, filled with immense energy and tremendous awareness.

The problem with desire is that when it has arisen—and even five seconds of entertaining desire is too much—you cannot do anything about it. Then desire will have to take its full course; it will complete its circle, and you will be carried away in its grip. Only in the beginning can you do something about it: burn the seeds of desire right then and there. When you identify the point of rising desire, then you can begin to separate from the urge and choose to go through relaxation instead. The response to go with our desires is a conditioned response, as if we flick into automatic-drive mode, so naturally it takes some practice and experimentation to steer away from the excitement track. After a while of separating from desire, the heightened feelings you experience will cease to translate into desire but will transform themselves into expansion and deepening of sensitivity. A little excitement in the beginning is always good to bring the body into excitation, but then there is a corresponding need to relax and allow the expansion of that very same energy through the system. In reality, desire and horniness are *not* prerequisites for sexual congress; in fact, more can happen when two bodies meet as relatively unexcited beings.

A woman shares her experience: "My husband and I decided to do an experiment with the clitoris without penetration. When he first touched me on my clitoris, it felt as if a button was pushed. As he touched me and moved his finger around my clitoris, I started to feel horny. I got hot; the previously slow and fine sensations and energy movements in my body suddenly changed. I started to move up against my husband's body with urgency. My breasts went out of my awareness. They seemed not to be at all important anymore. My focus was now totally on my clitoris. My vagina changed from relaxed and open to contracted and narrow. I got into a certain stress, started sweating. I moved faster and faster. I had the impression that I *had* to go toward an orgasm. My body felt tense and my vagina got more contracted. The contraction went even more up toward my stomach. I started using exciting words. It was a stress. I could not really feel my body as a female body anymore. The deep connection I could feel with myself was gone. The deep love I could feel toward my husband was almost gone. The connection seemed to be cut. Joy was gone. It seemed more like stressful work, like a satisfaction I needed to have, a clear goal. It had nothing to do with love or my heart.

"There was a point when I could not and did not want to go on. I asked my husband to take his hand away from my clitoris. I tried to relax my body, my vagina, to get back with my awareness to my breasts. I closed my eyes to return to the connection with myself and by that to my husband as well. I realized how difficult it was to relax my vagina. My husband and I then touched my breasts in a nice and soft way. By doing this I could relax more. But I could not really relax my vagina for a long time. It felt like cramps. This feeling stayed for hours. When we got together again with a soft penetration, it felt like a healing process starting from my breasts to my vagina and expanding to the rest of the body. I felt so good and connected again. My female part could start living again.

"We also did this clitoris experiment another time with penetration. My man did not have a real erection yet but he was inside me and it felt very nice. After stimulation of the clitoris it turned out that my contraction of the vagina got so strong (I would even call it horrible) that the penis did not have any chance to stay inside. It seemed it was kicked out. I am happy that we did these 'experiments,' as we have learned a lot. . . . I am not so ready to go for this experience of intense focusing on the clitoris again, as I know now that it hurts me on a very deep level; besides, my body does not like it anymore. I had not noticed this before. There is lots of very loving joy when we are together."

Tantric Inspiration

Excitement seems to be equivalent to ecstasy; it is not. Excitement is a state of tension; it feels good because the old is disappearing and the new is coming in. A new breeze, a new experience—it is good to welcome it with an excited heart. . . .

Excitement is only a welcome, but the welcome is not the whole story. Then the coolness has to come, and coolness is far deeper, far more valuable than any excitement can be. So jumping up and down has to stop. Sit silently, be calm and cool. Ecstasy is coolness, it is not excitement.

If you accept coolness, then only will the deeper experience of coolness give you the experience of ecstasy. It will be full of life, but not childish. It will be full of joy, but with deep contentment. The joy will not be against sadness, the joy will be beyond sadness.

OSHO, TRANSCRIBED TEACHINGS,
THE OSHO UPANISHAD

But excitement is not joy, it is just an escape from misery. Try to understand it very clearly: excitement is just an escape from misery. It gives only a pseudo experience of joy. Because you are no more miserable you think that you are joyous—not to be miserable is equivalent to being joyous. Joy is a positive phenomenon. Not to be miserable is just a forgetfulness. The misery is waiting back home for you: whenever you come back it will be there. When excitement disappears, one starts thinking "Now what is the point of this love?" In the West love dies with excitement, and that is a calamity. In fact love had never been born. It was just love of excitement, it was not real love. It was just an effort to move away from oneself. It was a search for sensation. You rightly use the word "fun"; it was fun but it was not intimacy. When excitement disappears and you just start feeling loving, love can grow; now the feverish days are over. This is the true beginning.

OSHO, TRANSCRIBED TEACHINGS,
LET GO! DARSHAN DIARY

Awareness and Sensitivity Exercise
Awakening the Secret Tantric Nerve

Give yourself twenty to thirty minutes on your own. At first it is suggested to do this meditation alone so that you can get the energy moving through the channel. Later you can use it as a kind of foreplay, as well as tuning into it while you are actually making love. You can also experiment with your partner sucking your upper lip, as suggested earlier in the chapter.

Lie down on your back, or sit upright with a straight spine. Visualize a subtle nerve running from your clitoris to your upper lip. You will be able to awaken it and consciously channel sexual energy upward through this nerve channel. From the clitoris, it runs upward through the center of the belly and chest to the base of the throat, and then through the neck to the occiput (the hollow at the base of the skull). Looping up to the crown of the head, then down through the center of the eyebrows, ending at the palate and the little hollow above the upper lip. It is like a serpent with mouths at both ends.

Visualize this nerve as an empty but vibrant tube, with a conchlike shape at the vagina/clitoris and a mouth at the upper lip/palatal region. Link some deep, slow breathing to a very gentle tightening of the vagina; this will awaken the nerve. Remember that strong contractions of the vagina during lovemaking can encourage male ejaculation, so be aware if you choose to do this, and do it very delicately so as to be almost imperceptible. Once you have connected with this path energetically, it awakens without any vaginal constrictions.

Partner Exchange Exercise
Exploring Excitation, Excitement, and the Full *Yes*

Give yourselves about forty-five minutes to do this exercise. Lie on your back side by side with your partner, with a space of about three feet between you and with no physical contact. Each of you take your awareness into your body and find a place of rest within yourself.

When you feel connected with yourself, slowly turn onto your side and face the other, allowing your eyes to meet in soft vision. After a few minutes, gradually move across the space that separates you. Place your hands on each other's genital area (one or both hands, depending on your comfort) as consciously and gently as possible, and fill it with your awareness and love. You'll find it extremely helpful in your exploration if you can report to each other in a few succinct words what you are experiencing in your body through the different kinds of touch. (See chapter 9 for more information about sharing the "now" during lovemaking.) If a certain touch arouses horniness, observe this, share it with your partner, and look to see how the touch can be modified so as not to create excess excitement.

You, the woman, want to avoid stimulating your man's penis, so don't do the usual masturbatory movements, with your hand copying the way a man would masturbate. Instead, hold his penis softly by wrapping your whole hand around it at first, and then a bit more firmly; then squeeze your hand and release it gently, slowly and lovingly moving up and down the penis squeeze by squeeze. From time to time simply hold still and embrace the penis with the warmth in your hands. With one hand you can also hold the testicles, firmly yet loosely, and delicately roll them around in your fingertips without squashing them in any way. Then hold the testicles with one hand and the penis with the other hand and melt into your hands, filling the penis with energy. Your man can very lightly rest his cupped hand over your pubic mound and follow this with a little tapping on the pubic bone and then resting still for a while. Then he can very gently pull one or two pubic hairs so as to cause a sensual little tug in the root of the hair. Again, he can rest his hands in a cup shape over your pubic mound. Continue for as long as feels right. The art is to create aliveness and excitation while bypassing overwhelming excitement that leads to desire.

8

Woman's Part in Man's Erection

We generally consider an erection to be necessary for sex, and we place the responsibility for erection exclusively on the man. With erection sex happens, without it sex is impossible—or so we think. At the same time, for a woman a man's erection is a delicate issue, and it can be an excruciating experience when a man does not respond with an erection, in spite of every loving affection. Easily a woman will take this personally, intuitively sensing that in some mysterious way she too is part of the erection phenomenon. But exactly how erection functions is not so clear.

Because sex is thought to be out of the question in the absence of erection, whenever erection *is* present every attempt is made to keep it up. The woman overcomes her insecurities by keeping the situation juicy and interesting for the man. She adds to the level of excitement by deliberately stimulating him or by getting excited herself, indirectly exciting her man. As we know, excitement in high doses will encourage—in fact, it will virtually guarantee—a man's early ejaculation. So when a woman actively assists with maintaining a man's erection through stimulation, she steps onto a tightrope. It is definitely in woman's best interests to prolong the sexual act and either prevent or delay her man from ejaculating. Lengthy lovemaking suits women because the more passive female body requires time for the sexual temperature to rise. By relying on excitement and stimulation, woman opens the door to premature ejaculation and suffers frustration instead. However, when a woman learns to be *more tranquil and serene* she can extend the lovemaking and also have a profound influence on male erection.

Woman Is Equally Responsible for Erection

We know that woman is the receptive element within the male-female dynamic, and this extends to the level of the vagina. Because of the equal but opposite polarities of the vagina and penis, exactly 50 percent of the erection response is an outcome of the environment surrounding the penis—the vagina itself. And really, when you think about it, this is as it should be: erection happens due to an interaction between the male pole, which is half of a circuit, and the female pole, which is the equal and opposite half of the very same circuit. When the magnetic poles are joined or lying within their spheres of influence, the poles exert a force on each other and erection is the outcome. The electromagnetic qualities of the male and female bodies build an erection through dynamic interplay. The positive male energy extends outward as it is simultaneously drawn inward by the negative female. This electromagnetic phenomenon makes the degree of femininity present, especially in the vagina, vital in determining true erection. The significance of this is enormous—a woman's influence on a man's erection is more profound than she ever imagined.

Thus, erection is not simply a matter of getting excited and staying excited. The presence of the opposite pole is required to trigger the mechanism in man. Excitement can be enjoyed for what it is—it is a choice we can make at any time—but it is important to understand that it is not the *source* of the male erection. The subtle electromagnetic properties of the penis and the vagina exist *beneath* the level of excitement, as an energy reality in the physical body. It is actually easier to perceive the interplay of opposite polarities in the absence of excitement, because with excitement the delicate deeper polarities are easily overridden and obscured. An erection that arises through polarity can be maintained for an hour or more without the usual efforts. An erection of this kind is a totally different sexual experience for woman and for man. It is like an inner earthquake that awakens every cell in the body. It is the most extraordinarily organic happening, full of the delicious sensations of the penis lifting and twisting its way into the vagina, writhing upward snakelike, touching woman to her very core.

Penetration without Erection

Because erection is possible at this delicate, organic level, we can begin to think about penetration (which usually requires erection) in a completely different way. "Soft" penetration offers us an interesting alternative style of lovemaking. It is very relaxing to begin penetration while the penis is soft. A woman can easily insert an unerect penis into her vagina, once she learns how. A man can also do it, but it is more fun all around when the woman actually puts the penis in the vagina—perhaps with a little help from the man, if necessary, who can join in holding the penis at its base. Often by this stage the penis has already started to respond to all the loving attention with the beginnings of an erection, and this makes the penis even easier to slip in. Soft penetration is a useful skill that, with a little practice, can be quite artfully done, thereby opening up a whole range of what hitherto were impossibilities.

With this new skill of putting the penis inside the vagina without erection, the lovers bypass the usual need for excitement or stimulation. This is an excellent way to begin intercourse, because it means the poles meet in a relatively undisturbed state, from zero so to speak. In the optimum scenario, of course, the woman has experienced an overflow, a showering of energy, onto her vagina from her breasts prior to the soft penetration; however, this is not absolutely essential. Quite okay, too, is to place the penis in the vagina after a short kiss and cuddle. Without excitement there may be a lack of lubrication in the vagina, and this is easily rectified with lubricants. (See more about condoms and lubricants in the partner exercise for soft penetration at the end of the chapter.) Once penetration is achieved, the woman can begin to bring her breasts into the foreground as elaborated in chapter 5, touching them, sensing them from within, or having her man touch them with love. And then it is a simple matter of waiting to see what wants to happen. In any event, the unerect penis can feel very delicious, and it is good to relax into whatever radiating sensations are present, *remembering that awareness at this level is what creates an environment conducive to erection.* A man is also able to sense his unerect penis, if not at first then certainly after a few attempts at diving into awareness in his penis. Most men in my workshops report that the penis is a great deal more sensitive by the end of a week, after being more conscious in sex.

In an unpretentious meeting of the vagina and penis, a natural kinetic of positive and negative follows from which erection can potentially unfold. I say it *can* because it does not always happen like this; it takes a bit of time for the penis and vagina to become accustomed to communicating at this level. On the other hand, it may happen on the first try! It really depends on the sensitivity of the individuals—and this will change at each moment and day by day. It is most likely to occur when a man and a woman are loving, intensely present, and relaxed in their general approach. Certainly when lovers achieve an erection in this way it is not by physical effort or fantasy. It is more likely a by-product of love, respect for the body, intimacy, and physical tenderness and is not something that should be expected *every* time. In this atmosphere the penis will naturally expand and wind upward and perhaps after a while relax and unwind. This is not cause for anxiety: if you wait without interfering, often the penis will rise once again.

In fact, starting out with soft penetration can be a tremendous relief to a man because it takes the immense pressure off him about *having* to achieve an erection before he can make love. This relaxation in itself helps his erection potential.

Healing Impotence and Lost Sensitivity

As explained in chapter 6, conventional sex causes the vaginal walls to toughen up and thereby lose sensitivity and receptivity. So on the first few occasions a woman may not feel as much of the delicate and divine vaginal sensations she is in reality capable of. Usually, though, she *will* feel herself and she *will* feel the penis in her vagina *before* the man can actually feel his penis himself. The penis, too, has become insensitive and overcharged, the tissues hard, tense, and dense. In this state of congestion it is very difficult for man to really perceive his penis without movement, let alone be a channel for his masculine force to flow into woman. So this lack of sensitivity is quite normal. But the good news is that relaxing together with the genitals in electromagnetic connection is a powerful healing force. The body responds very quickly and, depending on sincerity and the frequency of lovemaking, the penis and vagina soon begin to feel increasingly sensitive and alive to each other, whether erection is present or not. The unerect penis in the vagina is also a delight, and increasingly so as sensitivity is reawakened. Orgasmic states can happen as easily with an unerect penis as with an erect penis.

Impotence, the inability of a man to get an erection, is a mammoth problem facing men and women these days. Generally speaking, impotence can largely be attributed to the tensions, aggressions, pressures, heat, and excitement brought on by conventional sex. Man's dependence on stimulation and sensation means that with the passage of time he may eventually lose all capacity to respond as he slowly loses his sensitivity to himself and to his surroundings (woman and the environment). In addition, men frequently are disconnected from their true inner feelings, which include feelings of inadequacy and hopelessness, and repress them instead. Repressing feelings only makes matters worse. On top of the physical congestion is emotional turmoil and sexual confusion, and so a man can lose all potency.

Through soft penetration and the gradually returning sensitivity of the genitals, impotence really can be overcome. The healing of the penis and likewise of the vagina is something that can only be done together. Each needs the other half for healing energy to arise. In a relaxed atmosphere the penis (and the man behind it) is more able to perceive and sense the surrounding environment, which is the source of his erection. Healing impotence takes time and patience, communication and expressing inner feelings, and it can be done.

The key for a woman is to continually develop awareness within her vagina. Each time of making love is a new chance to dive deep within and feel the vagina from the inside; to start to perceive it differently and treat it differently; to imagine it as a receptive canal and will yourself to absorb and be receptive. It may take a few attempts to trust yourself, but the outcome will be sufficient encouragement to spur you on your way. This can be an ecstatic journey that lasts a lifetime.

Receptivity and Fear of Not Feeling

Women generally carry a great fear of feeling nothing—no interesting sensations in the vagina *at all*—if they relinquish the movements of conventional sex. This fear is something to be squarely faced, because behind the barrier of fear of inadequacy lies a world of feminine experience. All kinds of fears are instilled in us through an accumulation of insensitive sexual experiences; but now, in this loving, tantric context, a woman can let go and allow herself to receive man, allow herself to be healed by him and with him.

The more present and conscious a woman is in her vagina, the stronger the man's erection response is likely to be. Remember also that the breasts are the route to the vagina, so these must not be abandoned and overlooked in favor of the vagina. It's best to be aware of both places at once. If that is a bit of a stretch (which it will be at first), then choose the breasts as the focus of your awareness and trust that the vagina will respond. If the sensation in a woman's breasts are suddenly intensified, for instance when she or her partner touches them, there is often an accompanying surge of energy experienced through the penis as it rises and burrows deeper into the vagina. The same effect results through breast awareness itself, without even the need for physical touching. When a woman increases her intensity of awareness or begins to melt with the breasts and really enters them from the inside, it serves to encourage erection or even retrieve an erection.

Man, as he is now, is easily overwhelmed by woman (who is a bit "male," herself), and especially easily loses his fragile erection response when woman's sexual overtures seem more like hungry demands than gracious invitations. Man needs space to fall back into himself in order to truly realize his masculine qualities. And woman needs time to relax into her element in order to have the required alchemic effect on man. With our habit of taking action in sex, right now it may seem far from natural to relax and absorb; with practice and commitment it will soon begin to make all the difference to the sexual exchange.

Some emphasis is given to woman strengthening the muscles of the vagina, or using contractions or pumping the vaginal muscles during sex to squeeze the penis. Usually she does this with the intention of encouraging and maintaining erection. It will be most interesting for women who use this strategy to hear that in exactly the moment a woman contracts her vaginal muscles intentionally, men report that they immediately begin to sense that they are losing their erection. The moment a woman makes a demonstrative, positive, male-like expression, it has the opposite of the desired effect. The flow of energy between negative and positive poles is disturbed; suddenly the complementary component is absent, and erection begins to fail. The penis will begin to shrink back and both man and woman will feel it instantly.

A natural flow occurs when there is an ambience of vaginal relaxation creating space for the delicate, organic phenomenon of erection. And essentially, woman is the space in which everything takes place. When man feels this magnetic flow emanating from his penis, as if drawn out of him and absorbed by woman, it gets easier to change conventional ideas that sex equals getting excited and coming. When a woman is more feminine—poised and centered in herself, relaxed and receptive in her body, with awareness in breasts and vagina—it happens spontaneously, without thought, that male energy extends outward in the form of an erection, without great effort or great excitement. A spark jumps across the space and the bodies follow in unison. At a certain level of sensitivity it is possible to lie and be enthralled by the magnetic goings on of the penis snaking up and down the vagina for many hours with no movement at all. Remember: making love frequently enables the sensitivity to return and the electromagnetic finesse to develop between the penis and the vagina.

A man shares his experience: "Making love has become a part of my daily life and the fulfillment of my deepest longings. More and more I reach that incredible space of no-mind, of endless love, of inner expansion without boundaries, of great bliss. To me it still is a miracle, every day again. The wonderful thing is to be able to reach that space as a couple, but also alone. I can feel how the stillness and depth of that state of being infiltrates my ordinary life in a very subtle way. And I realize that I have become much more conscious about the moments when I lose contact with myself. And I can quite easily return back in and down. How can life be so easy? For me it has become a deep meditation to be together with my partner in this way. It nurtures my whole being in a wonderful way. The way I go back to my daily habits has changed. I feel much more connected with that still-point in me."

A man shares his experience: "I am learning to trust myself. Many of the things we have spoken about I have felt or done before sometimes, but I didn't understand or trust it. Simply to be there, naturally, waiting—this is very relaxing. I can watch what happens between me and the other. All the little fine movements of energy I don't normally recognize while I am excited—the excitement is what stops me from relaxing more and trusting in my energy. I have noticed that I don't have trust in excitement. There is always this fear of losing the erection. This does not happen when an erection comes out of a natural energy flow, by itself."

A man shares his experience: "Today I experienced the interactions of male and female energy. I always felt responsible for everything that happens in lovemaking, but at the same time I always had this feeling that it is not true—there is something else that creates the situation as well. Each day now my trust, acceptance, and relaxation grows. I begin to feel what happens on the other side for my partner, that something in me activates something in her, and this activates something in me, and so on and on. It is the feeling of creating something together, and the ability to receive love grows."

A man shares his experience: "In the beginning a lot of conditioning came up. It was going so far that I couldn't get an erection. But as soon as I found the door out of my mind, an erection was there. The process brought me back to myself. The more I can relax in lovemaking the more I feel my sex energy. When I notice I am outside of myself with my energy and I bring it back inside of me, the energy increases and spreads out in my body. The energy that wants to flow out of my penis, the pressure that wants to ejaculate—if this energy comes back to my body, it spreads out in my body and relaxes me very much. The fear of ejaculating early, all the tensions there—the pressure falls away if I can own back this energy. It's softening to my body; I feel myself fluid, like waves in the ocean. The more I relax, the more the energy takes over. Suddenly a wave of feeling, of energy, comes and moves my body, then it slows down and I feel a soft energy flowing out of my sex center toward my lover. This is combined with beautiful feelings in my belly. Then another wave comes and carries me away. There is no fear of ejaculating, no pressure—the awareness is not only concentrated in my penis."

A man shares his experience: "This approach strengthens me immensely, gives me trust in myself, gives me self-acceptance, freedom to express myself. It makes me feel more worthy."

A man shares his experience: "I see that most of the time I am outside of myself with my energy in making love. I'm a doer. I want to give pleasure, to satisfy. The first days I missed an orgasm—the feeling that lovemaking was incomplete, the urge to masturbate was there. While making love I have to be very aware—I come so quickly to the point where I ejaculate because the pressure is so strong. This is changing now. The more I bring my energy back to myself, having no ejaculation, the more I am myself. It makes me more and more sexual. The longing for my lover increases—to be loving, soft, gentle, more sensitive. Going into my mind I destroy all this. If I can stay in my energy all feelings increase."

A woman shares her experience: "We plugged in again last night just to charge our batteries, and just as I was falling asleep B. went 'boom' and kept on going while I slept. He said he felt high almost the entire night, in and out of sleep, and that it was a totally new experience for him. Naturally we plugged in again this morning and amazingly he kept right on going. It was beautiful to see and hear him talk about it . . . but I am just a tiny little bit envious. For some reason I have problems holding my presence within my body these last days. I was more relaxed these last two times—I am juicy all the time, even when we are not plugged in, and I enjoyed just being with my man in this relaxed atmosphere."

Tantric Inspiration

And while making love, forget about orgasm. Rather, be in a relaxed state with the man, relax into each other. The Western mind is continuously thinking about when it is coming and how to make it fast and great and this and that. That thinking does not allow the body energies to function. It does not allow the body to have its own way; the mind goes on interfering. . . .

Relax with the man. If nothing happens there is no need for anything to happen. If nothing happens then that is what is happening . . . and that too is beautiful! Orgasm is not such a thing that it has to happen every day. Sex should be just being together, just dissolving into each other. Then one can keep making love for half an hour, for one hour, just relaxing into the other. Then you will be of utter mindlessness, because there is no need for the mind. Love is the only thing where the mind is not needed; and that is where the West is wrong: it brings in the mind even there!

OSHO, TRANSCRIBED TEACHINGS,
THE OPEN SECRET

Partner Exchange Exercise
Soft Penetration

See Figures 8.1, 8.2, 8.3, and 8.4 for suggested positions for soft penetration. The easiest starting position is 8.1, in which the man lies on his side, facing the woman. The woman lies on her back, bringing her pelvis close to his. Both open their legs, and the genitals will be naturally lying opposite each other. Bring the genitals together and wrap the legs around each other. If the man is lying on his right side, the woman places her right leg between the man's legs keeping her knee bent and her foot resting on the floor. and brings her bent left leg to rest on his pelvis. This is called the scissors position because of how the legs interlock in scissorslike fashion. The

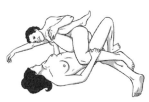

Fig. 8.1. Scissors side position for soft penetration

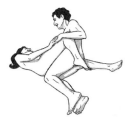

Fig. 8.2. Couple rolled to one side

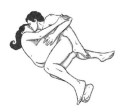

Fig. 8.3. Couple rolled to one side and kissing

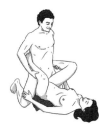

Fig. 8.4. Man in middle position for soft penetration

woman may have to move her upper body away from her lover's (to more of a 90-degree angle) in order to make the pelvises fit more snugly, or she can angle her own pelvis upward to the same effect. Experiment and find what is most comfortable (positions 8.2 and 8.3 make nice changes once penetration is achieved).

Once you are positioned correctly, pelvises close together and the vagina opposite the penis, the woman can now proceed. First take the penis in your hands. If you want lubricant, now would be a good moment to apply it. If you need a condom, now is the right time to put it on, while the penis is still soft. After the condom is on you can apply lubricant* and proceed directly with penetration as described next. Condoms do not interfere with electromagnetic sensitivity.

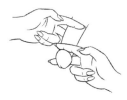

Fig. 8.5. Finger position holding penis for soft penetration

First take a moment to open your labia to make the vaginal entrance accessible. Then gently pull away the folds of foreskin wrapped around the head of the penis, exposing it even more while pulling the skin away and down toward the root. Next, make a two-pronged fork with the first two fingers of each hand (short fingernails to protect the vagina as well as the penis). Place one finger fork (try the left hand) firmly around the base of the penis and hold it there. With the other hand (the right hand) place the fingers directly on either side

---

*Use condoms only with a pharmaceutical lubricant, such as KY Jelly, absolutely not with a vegetable oil. Suitable oils for lubrication when no condom is necessary are almond oil, sesame oil, and olive oil. All oils and lubricants should be without perfume or scent.

and behind the rim, encircling the head of the penis (see fig. 8.5). Squeeze the fingers together so that you have a gentle grip on the penis and then pull the penis toward your vagina. When it arrives at the entrance, begin to insert it. You will be able to push the penis in and up into your vagina a little way. Release the fingers of your right hand and do the same thing again a little further down: grip the penis between your two fingers and direct it into your vagina, pushing it inward. By repeating the finger movement again and again, it is as if you're feeding or walking the penis into the vagina, gently pushing him inside a little more each time. Once you have pushed the penis inside you (or as much as you can manage to insert—even to get the head in is a good start), remove your hands, bring the genitals together as closely as possible by wrapping your legs around each other, and lie back. Use pillows for support anywhere you need them, and make yourselves as comfortable as you can. If the man tends to lean backward, wedge a pillow behind his pelvis and lower back.

You *absolutely must* keep your vagina relaxed during the soft penetration, or it will be like trying to force the penis through a closed door. It doesn't work. As you insert the penis, you most likely will want to look between your legs at what you are doing. Doing this will contract the belly musculature. When the belly contracts, so does the vagina. To avoid this tightening you will have to send your awareness downward into the vagina in order to intentionally hold it relaxed and open. The easier alternative, once you have the penis between your fingers, is to lie back for a moment and to stop looking at your hands. Then consciously relax the vagina and widen the vaginal muscles prior to attempting insertion. When open, slip the soft penis in, as described. Soft penetration can be a way of approaching lovemaking every time, or use it when you need it.

The scissors position may not work for every couple. In the middle position (figure 8.4) it is quite easy for a man to insert his penis himself—a good alternative. The man should position himself almost kneeling between the legs of the woman, who has her pelvis raised by a pillow. After pushing the penis into the vagina bit by bit (perhaps with the help of the woman), he can lie forward on her, and together they can roll onto the left or right side from time to time.

Tantric Meditation
Meditating on the Spine

You can experience this meditation lying on your back or sitting upright with a straight spine. Usually during sex, imagination is used to take the energy downward, but this pattern can be broken. The same imagination can be used to turn the energy upward. It can help to give the spine divisions according to the energy centers present in the body: at the genitals, below the navel, at the solar plexus, heart, throat, third eye, and the top of the head. These divisions can be used by the mind to help the energy move upward in fragments. If, however, you can connect with the spine as a whole, no divisions are needed.

Close your eyes, reverse your vision, and look back into your body, down into the pelvic area. Sense the bones of the pelvis and slowly bring your awareness to the sacrum and coccyx, which form the base of your spine. Visualize rays of light rising up your spine. Imagine yourself as particles of light, electricity. "Imagine your essence as light rays rising up your spine, from center to center, through the vertebrae, and feel 'livingness' arising in you."[1] Concentrate at first on your sex center and imagine that golden light rays are moving in an upsurge toward your navel center. Let the energy gather there and extend toward the solar plexus like a river of light. Feel warmth rising in you as rays begin to move up toward the heart center, filling you with warmth.

Travel gradually upward through your spine until you reach the top of your head. Feel your spine streaming from the sex center to the crown center. If you wish you can extend the connection beyond your body, imagining the light reaching about one meter above your head—and if you wish to travel further, reach out to the moon.

9

Relaxing into Orgasm

Relaxation, the foundation for new experiences, has many applications
and implications for a woman on the quest of regaining her femininity.
Relaxation creates an immediate aura of femininity around a woman. She
becomes porous, delicate; her whole being extends an invitation to man in
her presence.

The deep power in being a woman lies in her quality of being—in her
capacity to influence a man by responding to him from *within the female element.* From a place of receptivity, from poise, from rest and ease within herself she exerts a force on the space around her and on anyone who enters it.
She has the ability to transform her environment through receiving the male
force, be it by an embrace, a touch, a kiss, or penetration; to receive, drink,
absorb man as he penetrates her, with his touch, his body, his lips, his penis.
The more a woman can melt into her body and experience herself from
within, the more she will feel ecstatic. Relaxation and melting into the
moment become natural because there is no investment in a specific goal,
so an unhurried, easygoing interaction is possible. There is plenty of time to
perceive what is happening in the body as it is happening—to register it in
the depths of your being.

Pulling Awareness In and Down into the Body

The initial step for a woman in exploring the role of relaxation in lovemaking is to place the attention on herself. Her intention is to be more aware of herself and to be open to herself, to be curious about what is happening within. Without meeting herself in this way and passing through herself first, she cannot meet man in any profound way.

To relax means to pull your awareness away from the outside (and from doing), to pull it in and down into your body, to be awake in the senses, to feel your body's internal sensations and sensitivities. This requires a quiet atmosphere and a certain alertness—an atmosphere in which you have a chance to feel yourself rather than focusing attention on your man. To a large extent you are even ignoring your man. Not that you are oblivious to him; certainly you are not. You are vitally aware of his presence while holding the prime focus of your attention on *your* internal reality. When a woman begins to experience herself from within, she naturally becomes more still and receptive and immediately creates a feminine milieu around her. In other words, woman is required to turn her energy inward, not to project it. The true male (not the conditioned male, caught in hyperactivity) projects energy; he extends outward while woman moves inward, so as to be in a position to absorb male energy.

As receptive principle, woman is able to create a serene environment. Through relaxation she easily steps into her element and becomes an irresistible invitation. Her very presence invites the positive force and her desire is no longer a frustrated demand. When she learns to become an opening space, a fully present emptiness, she will experience that male energy is equally fully available to being received and absorbed, and transformed into something dimensional and completely fresh. In this alchemy between male and female elements an electromagnetic, attractive force arises. As a woman falls into the feminine principle the true meaning of sex dawns on her, and the real joy of being with a man begins.

Once the art is learned, she can exert her influence on any man she chooses. It is irresistible, magnetic, magical. A simple, sustained, lingering meeting of the lips can shake a man to his very foundation. Or a hug involving every cell in the body can last and last and last forever. Relaxation creates a kind of slipstream effect where man can effortlessly slide into place and connect with his equal and opposite. In my experience, man simply cannot maintain an aggressive, macho, goal-oriented stance when he meets a force that simply invites him to melt and merge through his body and penis. The presence and allure of the female body is tremendously amplified when relaxation is embraced in place of the physically strenuous activity normally occurring in intimacy.

Scanning and Sweeping the Body

There are many different levels to relaxation; it is a very subtle and multi-dimensional experience. On the basic level is actual physical relaxation. Habitually we hold many parts of the body tight without realizing it. Learn to scan your body continuously for unnecessary tensions. While embracing, while kissing, while making love, while moving or assuming any position, scan from head to toe and again and again relax any superficial layers of tension—consciously let them go. For instance, release the clench in the jaw, the tightness around the genitals; soften and let go of the belly and solar plexus; drop the shoulders a few inches; relax any curling at your toes and feet. Undoubtedly, a certain amount of tension is required to maintain any position in space; tension is a prerequisite for physical and bodily integrity. It holds us together. But we can drop all the extra tensions around that central tensegrity.

Sometimes relaxation is mistakenly interpreted as a sort of collapsed, absent, floppy doll state. This is a misunderstanding. Relaxation increases inner aliveness and vitality, it brings grace to the body and a radiance to the being. Relaxation is an attempt to make less effort; to start being, instead, more inner, more present to what is happening rather than chasing the idea of orgasm.

At a more subtle level, beneath this kind of immediate physical relaxation exists a deeper layer of relaxation that happens through employing awareness. Use awareness to filter through the body and to "sweep" through it, or to linger in certain areas, diving deep into the cells, becoming sensitive to the warm, tingling, streaming, glowing, vibrating sensations present in many places.

Delightful waves of inner expansion as well as a deeper level of relaxation follow this kind of lingering with the awareness, marked by a spreading of inner warmth and expanding sensations. Sensitivity becomes heightened. Body tissues get more porous as they are penetrated with life force. In particular, the vagina and breasts respond to such awareness, and a woman can greatly sensitize these two poles and thereby increase the magnetic flow between them. Inner awareness awakens the auto-ecstatic potential of the body through the magnetic rod—the source of orgasm (as explained in chapter 4). Essentially, relaxation implies presenting and opening oneself, not absenting and switching off to oneself. Woman can create an exotic ambience simply through expanding her awareness and being present throughout the slightest of any and all of her body movements and positions. Relaxation is a beautiful experience in that it finally allows a woman to be herself, present as she is, in all her glory, here and now. By adopting an easy, graceful attitude, not doing anything special, not going anywhere special, the enormous energy normally devoted to chasing the known pleasures of sex suddenly becomes free and available to expand into other areas. Instead of moving in an outward direction, the same energy is turned inward, rechanneled as it were, creating an intense awareness of the subtle, ecstatic cellular happenings within the body.

Relaxing the Vagina

Basically a woman should hold her awareness in the breasts as much as possible before and during sex, remembering that energy overflows from the breasts to ignite the vagina. At the same time it is good to ensure that the vagina is wide and relaxed. Linger with the awareness in the vaginal canal and sense into the tissues, entering them on a cellular level. Relaxation and sweeping with the awareness enhances the quality of "emptiness" of a receptive, welcoming vagina. This in turn reinforces the positive, active "fullness" of the penis present in the vagina. Once penetration has taken place the porous, absorbent, welcoming emptiness of the passive pole should be maintained for the duration of lovemaking. When these positive and negative poles are in balance (within your own body and between the penis and vagina), the passage opens, energy flows. The delight of this electromagnetic streaming within the core of the body is quite removed from the sensations we conventionally associate with sex.

Awareness naturally creates slowness, and so being unhurried becomes easy. Especially recommended are slow movements within the vagina to prevent an unconscious defensive reaction of the vagina as it attempts to protect the cervix. As mentioned in some detail in chapter 6, a tight, constricted vagina is a hindrance to orgasmic experiences. Instead of tight and narrow the vagina ought to be soft and supple, which immediately gives it the sensitivity to feel the energy radiating out of the penis. Encourage relaxation by keeping the vagina wide and open; there is no need to constrict or tighten it around the penis. The feeling of space and porousness is necessary for the electromagnetic qualities to be activated. When both poles are physically restricted, the plus and minus cannot meet, mingle, and interact.

Many women carry a fear of having a loose vagina with a widened channel after giving birth, but this is a misconception, a result of the conventional picture of sex. I was horrified recently to hear from a gynecologist that it is not uncommon these days for a woman to choose cesarean section instead of natural vaginal birth even when a cesarean is not medically required. Women are trying to bypass vaginal birth in a misguided attempt to preserve their supposed vaginal integrity.

Having mentioned the no-no's of intentionally flexing the vagina during sex, exercise of the muscles of the pelvic floor and vagina outside of sex is *highly* recommended as a means of maintaining the tone and health of the genitals and even of encouraging deep relaxation, as related in the exercise at the end of chapter 6. Exercising consists of consciously contracting and relaxing the pelvic floor, as if you were trying to stop the urine flow. Consciously done, these exercises will encourage an awakening in the muscular walls of the vagina, which increases the general tone and chi. They should not be done mechanically or absently, as this just creates hardening and insensitivity.

Combining Movement and Relaxation

To incorporate relaxation into the enjoyment of physical movements is an art—and a great deal of fun. In chapter 6 we considered the fact that when a woman moves her pelvis backward and forward, the very efforts of doing so contract the vaginal environment, usually making it less sensitive and receptive. With each forward thrust the vagina contracts and effectively squeezes the man out in the very instant he is trying to get in. This gives little chance for the plus and minus poles to meet, correspond, and exchange energies. As your man is thrusting I advise that you not thrust back. Instead, angle and hold the pelvis still, in a receptive position, and focus intensely on receiving the penis into the vagina. Also, encourage your man to make the penetration very slow, because this enables the vagina to be more available to the incoming penis. The slowness definitely highlights the delicious sensations in the vagina. If you wish, penetration can be sustained without an immediate reverse movement. As suggested in chapter 6, the optimum is to have prolonged minutes in the depths of the vagina before your man withdraws his penis and penetrates afresh. In this way your man reaches to your most receptive part, your garden of love, where divine, orgasmic sensations are contacted.

Not to contradict any of the above suggestions, movements back and forth are by no means excluded from the range of choices for a woman. Movement with awareness raises a whole different quality of perception in the body. It is not what you do but how you do it that counts—almost anything you do with awareness is going to be great. It is the lack of awareness that causes the obstruction. The main guideline is to avoid mechanical movements, as these tend to compress the body's energy and are usually done without inner feeling. This is how the connection to the inner world can easily be lost.

As mentioned, when a woman deliberately squeezes the vagina to stimulate the penis into erection, her action is slightly misguided. Erection is easily lost or ejaculation encouraged. Some techniques are a bit more advanced, for example when the woman attempts a pumping action with the pelvic floor muscles to push energy upward in the body. The amazing thing is that this kind of pumping action will in fact on occasion happen by itself. The body, given a chance to operate without our interference, does this from time to time. The body knows perfectly well how to respond with its own intelligence. (Perhaps the practice of conscious flexing of the pelvic-floor muscles originated as a mimicking of the body's response in the first place.)

While making love, sometimes just lifting the neck and head to meet the lips of the beloved is enough tension to introduce into the vagina, and this will increase sensitivity. Placing a pillow under the pelvis, as shown in the figures in chapter 6, is also excellent for creating an interesting tension in the vaginal cavity while keeping it receptive. Add these subtle tensions to kissing, and the interchange between the penis and vagina is wonderful.

Isolating and Relaxing the Vaginal Muscles while Moving

We can begin to think about movement in a few alternative ways. One way of moving is to change positions frequently without losing the contact between the penis and vagina. The penis-vagina unit is the central point around which all movements happen. (See figures 9.1 and 9.2 on the following pages for two sequences of positions that rotate around the penis and vagina.) When you want to move the pelvis, attempt to isolate the vaginal muscles and keep them relaxed and open while moving the pelvis itself. The pelvis is actually moved by a muscle in front of the spine (the iliopsoas), so when moving the pelvis, try to connect with that area behind the belly and in front of the spine. This is not so easy; it demands awareness. Check to see what other muscles are *not* needed for the movement (there are many, such as the buttocks, belly, and thighs), and be sure to use the muscles that *are* needed in a relaxed, slow, easy, conscious way. Slow movements guarantee awareness and increase sensuality. At times the two bodies will unexpectedly take off and move of their own accord in a rolling fashion as an outcome of the magnetic attraction and a circular movement of energy. Also, a whole range of reduced or smaller movements of the penis within the vagina are possible that do not result in much rubbing of the penis against the vaginal walls, and these are delightful to do any time or all the time.

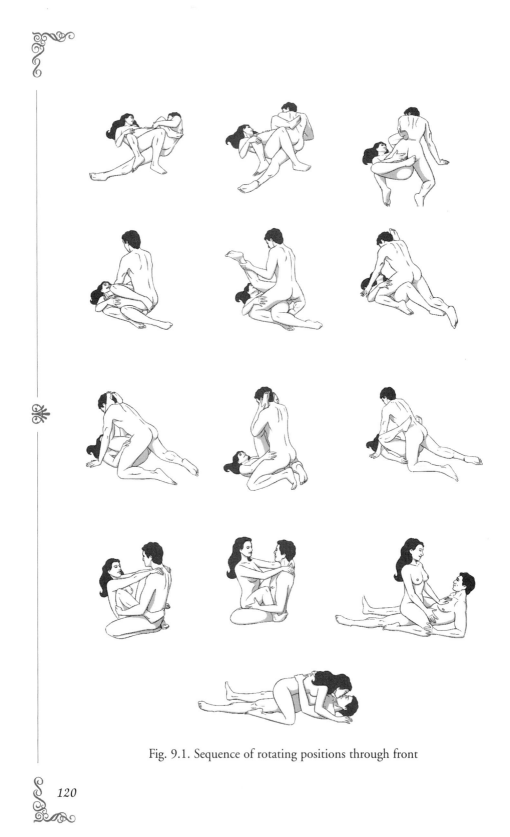

Fig. 9.1. Sequence of rotating positions through front

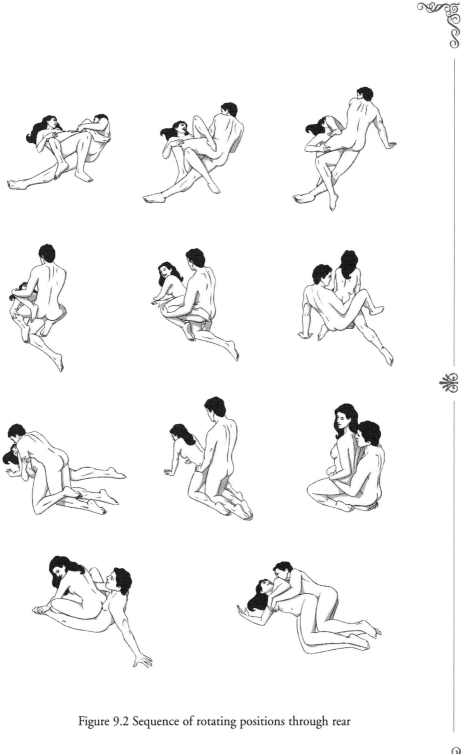

Figure 9.2 Sequence of rotating positions through rear

The essential thing to know is that tensions in general do not invite the deeper experience of orgasm, and can even work against it. In conventional sex there is a fair amount of activity and movement because we believe this is a prerequisite to sexual pleasure. But relaxation, not tension, is at the source of female orgasm as a prolonged, sustained state.

Using Breath, Words, Eyes, Lips

Relaxation hails the present moment, with nothing to do and nowhere to go. Lovers can greatly intensify the here and now in a few significant ways. They can use breath, words, eyes, kissing, and embracing all of the senses—each of these has an impact on the sexual exchange. Breath in itself is enough to lead to the orgasmic state. Breath keeps you in the present in your body, which is a good thing because you won't easily have an orgasm while you are in your mind thinking about something else. Breath helps you to merge with the body and become one with the source of life.

Ideally, breathing should be rhythmic, deep, and slow. Attempt to take the breath down into the belly; avoid taking it into the chest. Breathing through the nose is a more refined breath; however, breathing through the mouth is at times more comfortable or appropriate. Take the breath in the direction of the genitals to expand your sensitivity there.

You have probably noticed that, in practice, it can be extremely difficult to keep attention on the breath—especially while you are so involved with awareness on other levels. However, do return with awareness to your breath whenever it strikes you that you are not present to it. Consider your breath as a best friend that can help you out whenever you feel a bit less than alive and present. Breath always has a positive impact. If you are interested in pursuing the breath more deeply, it is helpful to create a balance between the length of the in breath and the length of the out breath. Count along with the exhale and the inhale for five or seven counts each way, or for whatever count suits you. With practice you will establish deep and regular breathing. Balancing the breath will also bring awareness to the moment between breaths, the *no breath*—a moment in which, floating ecstatically in the gap between the out breath and the next in breath, we glimpse eternal life. You can intensify the effects of the breath by using imagination too, which works wonders for some people. Imagine golden light streaming from the breasts on the out breath and golden light being drawn in through the vagina on the in breath.

Kissing brings a tremendous feeling of unity, in your own body and with your partner. When lovers' lips come together it is as if a circle has been completed, so the body sensations will intensify. Kissing helps a woman merge with her body. Kissing with the tongue penetrating the mouth easily leads to excitement, especially for a man, so it is a treat to be saved for rare occasions. But far more interesting than the tongue are the lips themselves. Keep your mouth closed and bring the lips together in a relaxed way. Infuse them with your awareness and then bring them into juicy contact with the lips of your partner, who with luck is doing the same thing with his lips. Make good, succulent contact, not a light and airy touch. Be as present as possible in your lips; imagine you are drinking from one another. I was touched in one workshop I led when a woman told me she and her husband had learned to kiss after twenty years of marriage. She was ecstatic about it—a new level of sensuality had opened up through the effects of truly kissing to her heart's content.

At times when you are not kissing, keep scanning with your awareness at the lips and mouth, because habitual tensions gather here very quickly. The habit is to pull the corners of the lips down. Experiment with this setting of the lips and pay attention to your mood; you will notice that you start to feel a bit miserable. Numerous people display this unconscious tension, especially women, because it is here that disappointment in life begins to reflect itself. To offset the drooping lip corners you can consciously raise your lip corners a few millimeters, into the tiniest hint of a smile. If you are observant you will notice an immediate sense of well-being: a contentment and a lightness rises up, lifting the face, and you may even experience the energy circling into the third eye area between the eyebrows.

Finally, speaking out loud what you are experiencing in your body is a way to amplify inner experiences immensely. Simply say what you feel and where you feel it. Start with the words "I feel . . ." and only talk about yourself, not your partner. The moment the words are spoken, your body will instantly respond with a spreading of the sensations already present. It is as if they answer to the acknowledgment with a kind of applause. We probably have all had the experience of putting a name to something and having a sense of ease follow. The same thing happens in making love. First, in communicating this way you are acknowledging your own body with your awareness. Second, sharing and speaking up has the benefit of informing your partner about what is going on for you. This in turn relaxes him because he doesn't have to guess. Through sharing in the sexual exchange, a man is able to learn from his woman what suits her and how it suits her.

"Sharing your now" means giving a short, concise report, a few words describing your inner experience. It does *not* mean having a long conversation about what is going on—on the contrary, the shorter the better. And you do not need a reply, although hearing your partner share *his* now in that moment, or any other, is wonderful. But if you turn a "sharing of now" into a conversation, you divert attention away from the intensity of the present moment, which leads to thinking and then, all too easily, to talking about old experiences that are not really relevant to the moment. The brief body reports help us keep track of what is happening moment by moment, without fantasy or imagination, past or future. Expressing tears or any feelings (again, simply) are also ways of sharing that increase body sensitivity.

A woman shares her experience: "Sharing so far has been the major key for me. From the beginning we shared anything that disturbed *the new*. As the sharing was mutual it helped me to drop all judgments and really share *everything*, which feels like a revolution. It makes me aware of the collective, and the depth of my conditioning—how much my ego, my self-worth is related to sex, to my pussy."

Communication is also greatly enhanced by the use of direct language; indeed, getting closer to one's own experience in sex, and that of your lover, requires the use of direct terms. For this reason I continually use the biological words *vagina* and *penis*. Often people will use more romantic or euphemistic words for the male and female genitals, like *yoni* and *lingam*, but this still keeps us in slight mystification and distance from ourselves. Experience has shown that it is helpful to communication to use the culturally accepted biological terms.

An event in a recent workshop in Europe may serve to illustrate this point. During the translation of my words from English into German, the translator (a man) twice used a crude but commonly accepted German slang word for the penis. On the third occasion of my using the word *penis,* I leaned over and whispered quietly to him, asking him please to use the actual German word for penis. It was difficult for him to do so the first time, and later a few times he made the same slip, quickly correcting himself.

On the final day of the group a man came up to me and said how important it had been for him that I had insisted that the translator used the word *penis*. He said that for him this marked the start of real communication with his wife. For the first time they were really able to talk about sex. Over the course of the workshop they became comfortable using a common and shared language, and so suddenly they could describe and share many small details, which before was impossible. When I shared this feedback with my partner, Raja, he said, "It's true, you know. You can say *penis* and *vagina* happily a hundred times over and over and it sounds fine, but for sure you can't keep saying *pussy* and *prick*. It just sounds wrong. Even *yoni* and *lingam* again and again is too hard." Unfortunately, many of the slang words associated with sex are degrading to women (and some are degrading to men as well). We would do well to slowly ease those kinds of words out of our daily expression.

The moment is also tremendously intensified if you allow a meeting of your eyes while making love. The eyes should be used in the way of soft vision as explained in the exercise at the end of chapter 2—no hard and fast staring, but a passive, receptive, inward vision. This inverting of the energy that is usually dispersed in actively looking allows that energy to fall back and flow onto the heart, opening it. Closing your eyes is also fine—it enables you to sense more deeply into yourself in certain moments—but keep them open as much as you can. The eye contact helps enormously in releasing old patterns of self-consciousness, being embarrassed by sex and the like. At first it can be challenging to be confronted by our limitations, but usually some tears or laughter, even a shiver or a shake, will do the trick and burn up our sexual confusions.

Women Sharing Experiences

"It is beautiful to keep eye connection. It makes it easier for my body and vagina to receive my partner. I experience energy moving from my eyes to my heart and from my vagina to my heart. I feel very good, very happy."

"I was a bit apprehensive about the eye contact as I have been used to keeping my eyes closed a lot of the time—but actually I liked the space it brought me to. It definitely added another loving flavor to the flow with my partner."

"I realize the importance of being *inside* first, centered in oneself before connecting, and then *staying inside* while connecting—the more the better. It's also important for me that I do not feel my partner 'coming out,' becoming disconnected to his own center. Then his desire can feel like a demand, a wanting. Feeling connected this way is a delicate space to get to. It requires practice when we are not so used to it."

"Something exquisite is happening for me. I often feel, as I look in my partner's eyes while we make love, that I am looking in the eyes of a Buddha. I thought such an unconditional love could only exist between me and my Master. Now it is right here."

"I find more peace in me. I discover my female side more and more. I feel this quiet happiness. I feel there is a healing process occurring on many levels. Old patterns come up once in a while, but as long as we stay open about them I can deal with them. The awareness of the eyes receiving images instead of looking outward helps so much to relax us. The energy is so different. We have not experimented so much with different positions yet, but we did experiment with small changes in one or two positions. It is amazing how a small change in a position or a small change in the movement can change the energy so much. How or where my lover is touching me is changing my own energy flow."

"We are very well, feeling happy and fulfilled, our love warm, tender, and wonderful. We're having fun experiencing more and more about lovemaking. For me it's mainly experiencing the expanding orgasmic waves up to my solar plexus/heart area, which feels so ecstatic when it happens. It's also great to feel that it doesn't matter if it doesn't happen because I can experiment again next time and again and again. It's a wonderful release to experience that lovemaking has become an important part of our lives and has gained so much priority. This helps me a lot to relax and just be with whatever happens. My man is still ejaculating often, but we stay together for a long time before he does. I am really improving being in the here and now and enjoying what is instead of looking for something else to happen. Sometimes, in lovemaking, it's like unseen doors are opening up, giving me deepest insight into questions I might have about life or death. It's like getting flashes of stunning clarity—comparable to experiences I've had in deep meditation. So it is wonderful, and I am very happy."

"I must tell you my wonderful progress. I have had my first truly wonderful orgasm with my man's penis in my vagina . . . with no pain! This has so far been unachievable in our twenty-three-year relationship! I still cannot believe how much has changed for us. We will keep going this way because it works—it is a healing process. It can change everything in the way we perceive ourselves and it makes us conscious in making love."

Letting Go of Tensions, Masks, Protections, Efforts, and Projections

As you can see, when moving into relaxation and opening up to the moment, the outcome is a great deal *less* tension and the dropping of masks, protections, efforts, and projections. What you gain is vitality, a physical porousness, and a psychological openness that expands the energy body. Orgasm always requires openness, so the tiniest bit of relaxation on any level, however achieved, is a good thing. As we know by now, relaxation is basic to orgasm, even a conventional orgasm. The orgasmic state tends to follow upon being more natural, dropping parts of our artificial, social selves. A woman often thinks that she is required to be open to a man before she even shows herself or can relax in sex or explore sex. But this is a misunderstanding. When people are open they are open *to themselves* first of all. By virtue of *their being* open, they open up to another person. So opening to ourselves comes first and foremost, and as we open up we become aware of the many unconscious tensions in the body: where and how we hold ourselves so tight. Many women's bodies are extremely hard to the touch, with contours that are not at all feminine. Tensions act as a subtle form of protection and defense against vulnerability. We fear an unloving reaction, based on previous experience. Even though these reactions may be absolutely valid in their own way, reimagining yourself, perceiving yourself from another angle, and opening into your femininity all require a vulnerability and healing of past wounds that is liberating and revitalizing.

A woman shares her experience: "I begin to love being present more and more, just as a means unto itself. I notice over and over again that I actually feel more satisfied after two hours of soft penetration than after a so-called fuck. Today I felt very horny twice and then realized I did not feel anything in my vagina; the source was absolutely in the mind. When the wanting comes, a key for me is to bring the energy back to the source of the wanting, and I am again flooded with energy."

To explore unknown territory always requires courage, but the rewards are huge. We step away from our inherited ideas to discover that simple relaxation is quite thrilling. It takes us far beyond the enjoyment of sexual pleasure by providing the possibility of sexual ecstasy.

The Difference between Lust and Passion

In doing research on sexuality I have found precious gems of insight along the way. One comes from Barry Long, the Australian spiritual and tantric master who has made an immeasurable contribution to returning men and women to their true, loving, sexual selves.* While he does not incorporate some of the polarity insights that are basic to the ancient tantric teachings (for example, he ignores the breasts), Long does give women a tremendous amount of support and inspiration. His specific guidance in sex is that a woman should remain very still and very present. And he uses the beautiful phrase "passionately undemonstrative" to describe the state to which women should aspire. At first glance these two words appear to be opposing, and an inevitable question pops up—how on earth can passion be undemonstrative? To us it may seem that passion is demonstration itself—the ultimate demonstration.

To understand fully what Barry Long is suggesting, we need to clear up our confusion about lust and passion and what these two states represent. Interestingly, Long says that "passion is pure presence." In conventional sex, when we are not present because of our interest in orgasm, most of us experience lust and mistakenly think it is passion. In reality, lust is linked to stimulation and excitement and somehow being out of control. Lust almost always has a direction and an end point. In contrast, passion is the experiencing of the intensity of the moment with inner stillness—not necessarily without movement! A highly passionate state can be stepped out of at any time in case of emergency (to take an important call, for example) without any "ruffling of feathers." But lust that is not completely satisfied will leave you frustrated and upset, more like a bird that just got all its feathers wet. Passion is not necessarily active or outgoing; it is a state of being in which every cell in the body is vibrant, flowering with life. When a woman becomes passionate she falls into alignment with her

---

*More than twenty years ago, Barry Long produced two audiotapes entitled *Making Love*. The revolutionary content on man and woman and sexual love has made a lasting impression on me and substantially furthered my personal journey toward demystifying sex.

inner body polarity, becoming utterly present in every cell, exuding an invitation but taking no direct action. This is the state of being passionately undemonstrative. In this state, a man is able to truly respond as man. When a woman is able to get herself into some semblance of inner "order," then a man can stop running around in sexual circles like a dog chasing its own tail. When a man experiences his energy being received by a woman, moving through his woman and thus through himself, his life is changed, something deep falls into place. He has been waiting for that moment all of his life.

While heeding and exploring Barry Long's insight, Osho says, "be wild, but do not become unconscious."[1] Notice that Osho's words warn against unconsciousness but certainly not against wildness. Wildness in this sense means a state of passionate wildness, not lustful wildness as we commonly experience it. He says that in that state, wildness is beautiful and there is nothing wrong in it; because the more wild, the more alive. "Then you are just like a wild tiger or a wild deer running in the forest . . . and the beauty of it!"

The Solar Plexus and the Third Eye

True passion arises in a woman through the solar plexus being open and free of hindering tensions. The solar plexus is a tremendous source of the love force and of genuine spontaneity. For this reason it is a highly significant area to become attuned to, connect with internally, and hold in your awareness while making love. For many people the power of this third energy center is blocked, through tensions from controlling, struggling with others, and suppressing feelings. (The negative effects of these will be covered in more depth in chapter 10.)

In much the same way, the third eye—the sixth energy center, situated between the eyebrows—has power in influencing the sexual energy to rise, although for women it should not be a point of extreme focus, especially in the initial phase of exploration. Far more important for woman is the connection to the breasts, the expansion at the heart center. From here the third eye (so called because its tissues resemble the retina of the real eyes) will open as a by-product. With the third eye acti-vated, a woman becomes a visionary and a source of true wisdom. In the awareness and sensitivity exercise at the end of the chapter are tips on how to connect internally with the solar plexus and third eye. These techniques can also be used while making love, amplifying a woman's internal experience.

Ecstasy Is Cool, Not Hot

For a woman with an inner openness to herself, sex becomes a cool expe-rience, even if it can get wild at times. Our ideas inherited from conven-tional sex leave us with the imprint that ecstasy is a hot, steamy, and overwhelming affair. But in reality, bliss and ecstasy engender the ultimate experience of coolness.

It is important to grasp that the word *cool* does not mean cold, with its negative connotations. *Coolness* is the experience of being rooted in yourself first and foremost. Eternal bliss is sometimes described by the enlightened ones as being cool as the eternal snow on the Himalayas. Certainly every blissful person I ever met was never hot and excited and jumping up and down all the time, but instead was wonderfully serene, inwardly composed, and simultaneously passionate and alive. To reach such a state of blissful passion might seem light years away; but any jour-ney can start with a few tentative steps. The key is to relax into oneself first. This naturally places woman in a more passive role, where she *responds* according to the polarity and does not *react* according to the personality. Being passionately undemonstrative produces a dynamic, attractive force that draws man toward you as you repose in body and being.

As we have come to realize, for orgasm to unfold and flower into a meaningful experience, a woman needs *time*—for preparation, for open-ing up—before the actual sexual exchange begins to appeal to her. The female body requires loving foreplay, with prolonged kissing of the lips, sensitive and featherlight caressing, and touching advances to awaken her yearning to make love. Real clock time is required, though when an orgasmic state arises one moves into an experience of complete timeless-ness. Five minutes can feel like five hours, and vice versa. The minimum time for lovemaking should be about forty-five minutes to an hour, and of course two to three hours is even better. Once in a while, take a whole day in bed, making love again and again and again.

In general, people think about sex more than they actually have it. When they eventually get around to it, it's over in a few short minutes. Many a woman perceives herself as frigid because she cannot open up so quickly to a man (and because some man has told her she is so). This is not frigidity. This is a natural reluctance to enter the sex act the way it is commonly done these days—as just another task in a busy day, without adequate preparation. If given sufficient time, women *love* to make love—especially when warmed up to a full-body *yes*.

In foreplay, much depends too on the intention and awareness of the *giver* of the touch or the kisser of the breasts, lips, and nipples. The inten-tion prowling behind the scene can be to excite and make horny and lust-ful. The opposite intention would be to love, to innocently say a sweet hello, to awaken from slumber. The role of foreplay is to energetically raise the octave in woman; however, when a man's intentions are loving, raising the woman's sexual temperature is *not* always an absolute necessity. You might embrace and caress for hours, or you might just "plug in" with soft penetration as explained in chapter 8. When lovers take the serene approach to sex and the man offers the famous "cool hand" to his woman, she will start to really turn on, perhaps even to her own surprise. As the woman melts into her female positive pole at the breasts, the man can focus on his own positive pole, in the perineum, central to the pelvic floor, rather than in the head of the penis itself. The energy then rises upward by itself. You do not have to concern yourself with the ascending energy: it happens without you. Your focus is in retaining the energy, not letting it leak out. A leaking pool has to be sealed before it can fill up. Both of you can relax, floating in that filling pool. Stay with it. Don't be tempted to pursue some avenues of excitement that send you racing off to the end.

Make a Date to Make Love

When you notice that there is a shortage of intimacy in your life, when daily commitments get in the way of your love life, when lovemaking ceases to flow spontaneously, then you need to intentionally make a date with your partner. Make special appointments to meet and dedicate your time entirely to making love—just like you make an appointment to meet a friend for dinner, or go to a party or to a business meeting.

This may sound a bit unromantic but it works extremely well. Each person comes prepared to make love, and it ceases to be an accidental happening. In time your lovemaking feels similar to two instruments tuning to one another, to create a beautiful piece of music. Bodies are indeed like musical instruments in that orgasmic states are created through fine-tuning and sensitivity. Mastering a musical instrument requires tremendous dedication and practice; in the same way, it requires lots of practice in making love to create ecstatic experiences until one gets the real hang of it. A musical maestro has to practice daily; if he doesn't he soon notices it, and within a few days his audience notices it. The more you make love, the finer your experiences become.

Tantric "quickies" are very much the order of the day when there is not adequate time to arrange a love meeting. Or, when it is late at night and you're a bit tired, plugging in for ten or fifteen minutes with soft penetration before sleep is a wonderful way to end the day. It transforms the rest of your day when you plug in before going to work in the morning. The beauty of the tantric approach to sex is that you don't need heaps of energy to make love; neither do you have to feel horny or sexually charged—you don't go that long without making love. Instead, you begin to have sex as a matter of course, just as you have dinner and breakfast. Love is essential food. There is no need to wait around for lust to overtake you. Many women begin to feel the failure of lust in their lives as they get older and think that their sexuality is failing them. They don't yet recognize that excitement cannot last forever and that coolness and relaxation can take its place. It's pointless to long for or look for the former signs of the strong, fierce sexuality you experienced when you were younger. You do not even have to really "feel like" making love; if you go ahead and open yourself and your body to love, in so doing you will receive endless love.

More Women Sharing Their Experiences

"Something new occurred in making love. It happened to me twice in the last weeks. When we were together, with very little and slow movements, orgasm came, and it felt completely different from the orgasm that I knew before. I ask myself if it is vaginal orgasm and if it is the orgasm that comes by itself when the body likes to orgasm? It was very soft, nonexciting, quiet. Afterward I felt filled up with new energy."

"Lovemaking has started happening, really in the sense of generating love. Also, my pleasure and my physical sensations are very strong. I am aware of this border between voluptuous space and sexuality—any small 'breaking of the rules' immediately brings a different space, and changes the union experienced before."

"I was totally in my mind and thinking during lovemaking in the afternoon. I felt that my husband was moving too slowly because I was wishing for the old release, but after a while my usual approach did not work—my husband tried it but suddenly I realized that I did not want it.

Then I told him my feelings, that I did not want to continue looking for an orgasm, and told him that I wanted to now go inside, so I closed my eyes and did so. All this time we were in penetration. When I came back we looked in each other's eyes and for a few minutes he slowly, slowly moved his penis inside me. I had an explosion of energy, in the vagina first and then very soon after that in the head. It was another dimension of energy. I think it was an orgasm, but not of a sexual quality—it was one from another world. I cried intensely and then I was laughing. At first my husband was confused and then we were totally together."

"We decided to sit in silence for a few minutes after making love, and that was great—the energy turned in again and I felt very silent and centered."

"My *aha!* of the day was when I realized that 'presence' in itself brings a feeling of total well-being, even ecstasy, even though 'nothing' happened, even though there was tension and an intense burning in my vagina, even though my partner was freaked out. So nothing was perfect. Still, I experienced such a feeling of being present. The eye contact, the breathing, the awareness of my vagina, of the birds outside, of the river. Everything became perfect with my acceptance."

"In my relationship we've both always wanted to move somewhere else with our lovemaking, but we didn't know how. There's a part that's delighted and another part that is scared, but we both don't want to turn around and go back to the old. It is very beautiful and very fragile."

"The more I relax inside the more I encounter a sudden feeling of lovingness—it comes and goes and has nothing to do with personal/psychological stuff—it is not emotion. It has nothing to do with me."

"This is the first time I've touched that part of my body. . . . I can feel my pelvic floor, my ovaries, my uterus from the inside—there is so much more space."

"We are having a very good time. After meeting with you I started to understand lovemaking on a deeper level. There was much more relaxation and I was no longer waiting for 'ecstatic energy things.' I started to see making love as another form of meditation, relaxation, and regeneration, not as a means for having 'super sex.' Now we enjoy all kinds of sex as it is expressing itself right in the very moment."

"We are well and happily making love. Our lives are going in different directions in one way, as my work is so different from my partner's and I am away a lot. However, having our regular dates for lovemaking, which we give just as much priority as anything else, it doesn't seem to matter. It is a rhythm of being apart and being together that feels very good, and it is a great experience for me. My man tells me that it is great for him too. This being together in love makes such a lot of difference! It leaves so much room for other things that we don't share without making us feel we are drifting apart.

"Lovemaking sometimes seems to me like it is about experiencing the full range of living life. It's the process of unlearning so much, of just being and experiencing whatever is happening at this very moment. It is so interesting to observe what happens when I am in my mind, entertaining concepts about how things should be or should not be versus when I am just fully present to whatever there is, loving every moment of it. Lovemaking like this is like a life school for me, and I am learning a lot by shifting my focus from 'shoulds' or 'should nots' to paths of fun and ecstasy. This has a strong effect on my work and on my whole life, which in return enhances the quality of our lovemaking. So it's just great."

"Even though in my mind I knew already that I did not have to please my man, I noticed that wanting to please still came up at times as a subtle pressure in my body. It showed itself in slight tension and a loss of energy sensations, and after some time even in not being interested in sex at all. This brought me into a deep insecurity and the feeling of being dysfunctional. For me it has been very important to have support from other women who have already been through these issues, which encouraged me to find my own truth—maybe it is even better to say 'to trust the truth of my body.' When I began to see the start of lovemaking as a soft, relaxed, and curious search for the entrance into a delicious and beautiful love garden instead of an effort to 'come into my energy,' things changed. It was no longer my responsibility to find my sexual energy to make my beloved happy. It became more like a journey together through a labyrinth, and the guide is my body. Both of us—my beloved and I—don't know where the entrance is today, because there is no recipe and it can be somewhere else every day, the way in can be new every time.

"Sometimes we find the way in, sometimes not. But if not, it is no longer my 'fault' for not being sexual enough. There is mystery to finding the 'magic word' to open the door. And to find this entrance it becomes totally important to listen to every little sign the body gives—to feel whether any touch or movement or even any thought is opening me up or closing me down and to dare to share this with my beloved, sometimes with words and sometimes with body language. It is beautiful if the man is able to surrender and let himself be taken by 'the hand' of the woman's body, so that the woman's body is allowed to be the guide for both. But if this is not possible for him, or if he is disappointed, I think it is important for the woman to go on trusting her own body and not to compromise. For me this way of love-making is still not easy all the time, but I definitely feel it this is the right way for me."

The Role of Relaxation

Not to be underestimated, relaxation is pivotal in woman's searching for satisfying orgasm. It is the real experience of sensuality as consciousness begins filtering through the body. The energy usually *ex*pressed turns inward and becomes *im*pressed. It sinks into the body, into oneness with the senses. Touch, sound, breath, eyes, hair, silky skin—all of these speak to us when we are relaxed enough to listen.

When a woman relaxes into herself, the adventure for a man is as momentous. A man needs only a couple of experiences to confirm how naturally the male energy responds to the presence of a complementary passivity—the sheer delight to be found in being welcomed, received, absorbed, and expanded through woman. Mistakenly, man has helped to make woman more male through his insistence on excitement. Yet ironically, man's sex obsession is a search for this very dynamic experience where his energy simply moves through him, drawn by an equal and opposite force—and both are fulfilled.

If you are single and without a regular partner with whom to make love, experimenting is more difficult—but not impossible. While you are making love, even if it is the first time with a new partner, just try a key practice. It might be bringing awareness to your positive pole, or slowing down. Or you may like to look into his eyes. How does he respond? It is very interesting to see what happens! If you continue to meet again to make love it is good if you can explain to the person that you are interested in experimenting with making love. Tell him a bit about how you feel and what you would like to experience. Again, it does help if you are on the same wavelength. Sometimes it simply doesn't work to talk about it—perhaps you don't even speak a common language, in which case just try relaxing into sex, experimenting on your own. Notice what works. Notice what happens. Keep bringing in awareness.

Tantric Inspiration

Many people would like to relax, but they cannot relax. Relaxation is like a flowering: you cannot force it. You have to understand the whole phenomenon—why you are active so much, why so much occupation with activity, why you are obsessed with it.

Remember two words: One is "action" and the other is "activity." Action is not activity, activity is not action. Their natures are diametrically opposite. Action is when the situation demands it, you act, you respond. Activity is when the situation doesn't matter, it is not a response; you are so restless within that the situation is just an excuse to be active.

Action comes out of a silent mind—it is the most beautiful thing in the world. Activity comes out of a restless mind—it is the ugliest. Action is when it has relevance, activity is irrelevant. Action is moment to moment, spontaneous. Activity is loaded with the past. It is not a response to the present moment, rather, it is pouring your restlessness, which you have been carrying from the past into the present. Action is creative. Activity is very destructive, it destroys you and it destroys others. . . .

Remember, activity is goal oriented, action is not. Action is an overflowing of energy; action is in this moment, a response, unprepared, unrehearsed. The whole existence meets you, confronts you, and a response simply comes. The birds are singing and suddenly you start singing—it is not activity. Suddenly it happens. Suddenly you find it is happening, that you have started humming—this is action.

OSHO, TRANSCRIBED TEACHINGS,
TANTRA: THE SUPREME UNDERSTANDING

Awareness and Sensitivity Exercise
Activating the Microcosmic Orbit

Give yourself half an hour or more for this exploration. You can do this exercise sitting upright in a chair with a straight spine and both feet on the floor.

Close your eyes and tune in to two energy channels, or meridians: one running up the back of the body and the other down the front of the body. The channel at the back begins at the perineum, between the anus and the vagina, and runs up the sacrum and low back, up the spine, over the top of the head, to the roof of the mouth. The channel at the front runs from the tongue down the throat, heart, solar plexus, and navel, to the perineum. When these two main channels are open, the energy will circle automatically in a loop that Mantak Chia calls the *microcosmic orbit.*[2]

The tongue is the bridge that connects the yang male energy channel along the back to the yin female energy channel along the front. Place the tongue on the soft palate at a point toward the rear of the mouth cavity, about one and a half inches behind the teeth. It is a slight stretch for the tongue. (Closer toward the teeth is okay too, if the suggested tongue position is not comfortable.) By completing this route you get the yin and yang harmonizing, enabling you to increase the energy flow and vitality throughout your body. The direction of energy flow can also be reversed—moving up the front and down the back.

To awaken the energy at individual points along the way, use your inner vision. Attempt to sink your mind into your body, to the point you wish to activate, and soon you will feel warmth or energy or chi beginning to flow there. Each person will experience this energy activation differently; just stay attuned to your sensations in the body. The best place to start the circle is by focusing deep into the navel, and from there flow downward to a point just above the pubic bone (a point corresponding to the ovaries), then to the perineum, the coccyx, the lower back (on the same level as the navel), the mid back (on the same level as the solar plexus), behind the back of the neck just where it joins the head, the crown of the head, the point between the eyebrows, the tongue/palate, the heart, the solar plexus, and returning finally to the navel. Concentrate on the energy points and circling the energy; it is not necessary to focus on the breathing.

When you are finished, always complete the circle at your navel center and store energy there. To store energy, place your right fist on your navel and concentrate your attention there. Rotate your fist counterclockwise thirty-six times in an increasingly large circle, then reverse the direction, rotating clockwise twenty-four times while shrinking the circle back to the navel. Allow a little smile at the lip corners during the whole exercise, and notice the feelings of harmony and love. Rest for five to ten minutes after finishing.

After you get the feeling of this circle, you may hook up with it any time you are making love, to great effect. It is especially nice in yab yum, where you are in a sitting position and in line with Earth's gravitational field.

Awareness and Sensitivity Exercise
The Solar Plexus and the Third Eye

While you are making love—or any time, as a matter of fact—it is possible to intensify the focus on the solar plexus area by looking down to the point of your nose, which will give the sensation of the eyes crossing. Holding this eye position for a few moments enables you to sense into the solar plexus very deeply.

To help activate the third eye, between the eyebrows, almost close the eyelids and then start flickering them up and down very quickly *while at the same time* looking upward, directing your eyes toward the center of your forehead. Again there will be the sensation of the eyes crossing. Gradually look back as far as you can without strain. After a few attempts at this you will begin to get the sensation of something locking or converging in the area between the eyebrows. Close your eyes and continue to hold awareness at the third eye—the sensations at this energy point will be greatly intensified. You may only be able to do this for a few short seconds at first, but that is a good start.

Try these two practices on your own first before trying them during lovemaking. You can actually do them in sequence, looking down to the solar plexus, then looking up to the third eye a few minutes later, then down again and up again three or four times.

Circling energy through the microcosmic orbit, or lifting the lip corners into an inner smile, or simply placing the tongue on the soft palate, or connecting with the solar plexus or the third eye—the stimulation of all or any of these energy phenomena even just for a few seconds will have an impact on the sexual experience, and can be utilized at will during lovemaking.

Partner Exchange Exercise
Let Lovemaking Come by Itself

Before you move into love, sit silently together for fifteen minutes holding each other's hands crosswise. Sit in darkness or very dim light and feel each other. Get in tune with each other by breathing together: when your man exhales, you exhale; when he inhales, you inhale. Within a few minutes you will get into it. Breathe as if you are one organism—not two bodies but one. And look into each other's eyes with soft vision.

After fifteen minutes, take time to enjoy each other and play with each other's bodies. Don't move into love unless the moment arises by itself—not that you make love but suddenly you find yourself making love. Wait for this—do not force it. Go to sleep—there's no need to make love. Wait for the moment to arise even if you wait two or three days. It will come, and when it does love will go very deep. It will be a silent, oceanic feeling. Love is something that has to be engaged in like a meditation. It is something that has to be cherished, tasted very slowly so it suffuses deeply into your being. It becomes such a possessing experience—as if you are there no more. It is not that you are making love—you *are* love. Love becomes a bigger energy around you; it goes beyond you both.

10
Mastering Love and Overcoming Emotions

What is love? Love is the fragrance, the radiance of knowing oneself, of being oneself. . . . Love is overflowing joy. Love is when you have seen who you are; and then there is nothing left except to share your being with others. Love is when you have seen that you are not separate from existence. Love is when you have felt an organic orgasmic unity with all that is. Love is not a relationship. Love is a state of being. It has nothing to do with anybody else. One is not in love, one is love. And of course when one is love, one is in love—but that is an outcome, a by-product, that is not the source. The source is that one is love.

OSHO, TRANSCRIBED TEACHINGS, *THE GUEST*

As we now know, tantra sees human energy in terms of polarity: feminine energy as "being" and masculine energy as "doing." Within woman, the inner masculine is active, logical, and result-oriented; while in man the inner feminine is receptive, intuitive, and process-oriented. Tantra takes a step further to say that the highest spiritual polarity in existence is love and meditation, that woman embodies love and man embodies meditation. This implies that woman's inner man is meditative and man's inner woman is loving. To be whole human beings, operating with wisdom, passion, authenticity, and spontaneity, we need to master both energies: masculine and feminine, meditation and love. Woman gets more meditative the more she loves and man gets more loving the more he meditates. In more precise sexual language, to love in woman means to welcome the penis in and surrender to its power. And to meditate in man means to merge with and become utterly present in his penis, inside woman, in stillness.

Distinguishing between Emotions and Feelings

Yet for too many of us, deep personal and societal wounding through sex prevents us from balancing our energies in a way that serves us. We repress the memories of our hurts, suppress our real feelings and energies, and then unconsciously begin to control or manipulate others or fail to channel our energies in a wise or creative direction. As we change the way we make love, we initiate an alchemical process of awakening the inner opposite polarity within, which in time enables us to use both energies powerfully and productively. This, in turn, helps us to dissolve the emotional patterns that have caused us pain in the past and to create the life and love we deeply desire in the present.

To create the life of sustained loving harmony that so many women desire, an important step to take is to keep emotion out of love. As Osho says, "love is a state of being," and "one is not *in* love, one *is* love . . . it has nothing to with anybody else." With the new input about harnessing polarity and female orgasmic potential, you might be able to conceive of a day (or at least a few hours at a time, a few days of the week) of *being* love as a state that is sustained and not associated with the highs and lows of relationships. But these highs, and the painful and difficult lows filled with emotions, where love becomes scrambled up with irreconcilable feelings and fears: what is all this about? Despair or resignation can set in when a couple can see no way out of the cycle of conflicts.

Regaining female power is dependent upon knowing the difference between feelings and emotions, and knowing that "love has to be separated from this category of emotions." (See the tantric inspiration at the end of this chapter.) The crucial understanding here is that emotion comes from the *past*, while love and true feelings arise in the *present*. When too much past stuff gets dragged into everyday life, love is quick to wane. Love has its tendrils in the delicacy of the now. That doesn't mean that you should think of emotion as some kind of demon. Emotion itself is fine; what is important is that you are *aware* that you are emotional, that you know what is happening when it is happening. This understanding changes everything.

Symptoms of Emotion

Until now we have had no frame of reference to understand what is truly going on in the split second when emotions surface, the instant when, out of the blue, the love boat begins to rock dangerously. What we need is self-awareness. The immediate physical symptoms of emotion can be described variously as "suddenly feeling paralyzed," or as if "a wall suddenly comes down," or as a moment when it is impossible look the other in the eyes, or having the awkward sensation of feeling disconnected from everything, utterly separate, lonely, totally misunderstood, physically collapsed. Often we find ourselves full of vengefulness and wanting to hurt back. We start blaming our partner for the situation, using the accusing words "You never . . ." or "You always. . . ." Or, alternatively, a jumble of feelings tumble around inside that are impossible to find words for. When one of these types of "emotional attacks" takes place, we must recognize that emotion is in play. It takes some practice to recognize emotion, but after a while it does become obvious.

This inner acknowledgment immediately puts things more into perspective. Emotion is, in reality, the resurfacing of an accumulation of old feelings, repressed feelings, feelings that had to be swallowed, that we did not dare to show or express *at the time* when the feeling was actually taking place—in a previous present, during some unhappy incident many years ago. This is why so often emotional reactions are quite disproportionate to the slight comment or mild action that triggers the emotion. The trigger itself does not usually warrant the huge upset that follows in its wake. What is really happening is that old, unexpressed feelings begin to resonate and bubble up inside and create confusion. When you acknowledge these old feelings for what they are and work their negative effects out of your system, emotional reactions will begin to cease. In a few years your partner can say precisely the same words to you, and nothing happens—the comment slips by you like water off a duck's back.

Using Love to Overcome Fears Created by Lack of Love

As women we carry many emotions, which means we are loaded with layers of unexpressed feelings. The source of unhappiness is most usually due to a lack of love, perhaps to abusive and hurtful sexual experiences of the past, where there was a total absence of respect and love. Even if a woman has not been intentionally abused, the current style of aggressive, insensitive sex can be acknowledged by a woman's body as a subtle form of abuse. This implies that basically all of us are emotional about the lack of love, not only in the past but perhaps even now. Deep fears are instilled by the unloving treatment that negatively affects a woman's capacity to love and be loved. Fear demands the need for protection and defense, so it is with good survival reasoning that woman protects herself from man.

However, to heal the existing situation and bring it back into balance (within us and between us) there is only one option open—if lack of love instilled fear, love is the direct method to dissolve the fear and thereby end the patterns of emotionality. A woman must trust her nature and allow herself to be loved by a man and open up to him (provided he is willing to be conscious in the tantric way), which means dropping the defenses, games, and emotions that form our personality but have nothing to do with the vulnerable sensitivity of our true selves.

The truth is, from our earliest years we have been developing feelings of being separate, of being wrong, of being unworthy, of not being good enough. We, who were manifested on earth as an expression of unhindered energy, become separate from ourselves, from each other, and from the whole of existence. As we cut off from our pure energy we also cut off from our *love source,* and gradually a false self develops around us as fear replaces security and joy. The fear is due to imprints made by an absence of love in the immediate surroundings (family and parents), and the fear provokes a child into acting differently in order to try to get approval (or disapproval, through rebellion, where at least some attention is gained) in order to gain the love so necessary for survival. And so our parents begin to write the script for us, for who we are and how we should behave, and we gradually lose our authenticity.

Emotionality is an unconscious, automatic reaction to a situation or circumstance, like when a switch is flicked off and light turns to dark. It can even be a learned habit: some women learned to be emotional as young girls by mimicking their mother's behavior. As the years go by, we as women begin to define ourselves according to our emotions, our little and big ups and downs, thinking this is who we really are. It is as if we are in a movie and the situation is not actually real. Only the past makes it real. (If we were to wake up one morning without our memory, with no past, what then?) But in spirit and essence we are all love, and to keep love alive love has to be separated from the backlog of stored emotions we are not so aware of. As we begin to release these old feelings consciously (whenever we notice they arise) they cease to hold our energy down.

The Solar Plexus and Emotion

In addition to the emotional alarm signals, like suddenly feeling paralyzed or disconnected, you can learn to recognize states of emotionality in the solar plexus. Consider this area as a sensor for recognizing emotion, because this is where emotions will gather and create a lot of discomfort. Emotions try to seek discharge in various ways—through irritation, complaining, nagging, passing on your frustration to the children. When you develop awareness of the solar plexus, the moment someone says something that strikes an uncomfortable chord in you, you will notice something going on there telling you that you are emotional, that something unresolved is being triggered. For woman it is good to have the solar plexus free of tensions to allow for unobstructed flow of sexual energy between the breasts and the vagina.

Many women will feel nauseous when first relaxing into lovemaking, but this is nothing to be concerned about. It is a sure sign of the surfacing of old feelings asking for release. Nausea is a by-product of the sexual energy expanding and pushing the restricting emotions out of the body. An ancient tantric technique is to drink a large amount of salt water and put a finger down the throat to open the solar plexus and keep it open. Even the vomit reflex alone, without any discharge, works wonders in releasing tensions of the solar plexus. There is an immediate feeling of expansion, as if something toxic has left you.

Verbalize Emotion, Separate, and Physically Move the Body

The very moment that you recognize that you are emotional, through the solar plexus or in whatever other way you recognize it, the first step is to inwardly acknowledge that you are emotional. The second step is to say it out loud to your partner. "I am emotional." This verbalization instantly brings a touch of relaxation, because at least now your partner knows that *you* know that *you* are emotional, which takes him out of the picture and no longer makes him responsible for your unhappiness. It is a difficult step to take, to admit you are emotional by actually saying so, because the ego will be fighting like crazy trying to blame the other. But in reality, until you take yourself back to yourself and acknowledge the past, your love life will remain a series of good times followed by bad times.

In such circumstances, having said the words "I am emotional now" to your partner as gracefully as possible, physically leave the room, adding the words "I need some time to myself and will return soon." Close the door gently and go outside or to another room in the house and take some time alone. (Do not drive off and feign that you are abandoning the relationship in that moment.) This is not switch-off time, but the time to switch on and release or get in touch with these old feelings residing in your system. In fact, when emotions get activated they move through a layer of connective tissue in the body called fascia. This explains why sometimes at the onset of an emotional attack you will feel that onset in your body very clearly, almost as if a substance with density is swirling through the body. (Indeed, fascia does weave dimensionally through the body and from head to toe about five times, connecting the superficial layers with the deepest physical layers.)

Now, to get rid of these emotions you need to help them out of the body where they are stored. It is essential to physically move your body so that the old feelings can be burned up. Be active in some way: hit a pillow, bang on a drum, jog, chop wood; if you are able to have a good scream that also helps, but that depends on your neighbors and your level of privacy. Gibberish nonsense talk also works to release emotions. Have a little catharsis—be crazy for a while! Whatever you do, be active. This is not always the easiest choice because emotions leave us feeling collapsed and exhausted and more like curling up in bed to nurse them. The surprising fact is that when you return to your partner after physical release you are likely to experience that the sense of separation/disconnection is reduced, that you can make eye contact, that the wall between you is crumbling. If this is not the case, then another bout of body movement is called for, until the wall has crumbled to the ground.

This sounds almost too simple, but it works. And it certainly wins hands down over the alternative option of dragging the emotions around for a few days, heavyhearted and miserable, wondering what has become of love until eventually, sleepless nights later, one side breaks down into tears, gives up the fight, and starts to express the feelings lurking behind the emotions. You have experienced this yourself many times, I'm sure: the very instant one side gives up and starts to express inner feelings the fight is over. We pick up the remaining threads of love and start again.

A woman friend who uses body catharsis through chaotic movement as a meditation has shared this with me:

> I continue to marvel at how cathartic movement frees a lot of my psychological holding, a certain mental rigidity that collects and periodically builds up through the activities of my day-to-day life. As a result of movement catharsis, I find I have more patience and focus in dealing with all aspects of my life. In addition, I find that cathartic movement is especially complementary to my yoga practice. I love practicing yoga, but there is something serious and rigid about it that wild dancing movement seems

to free up and balance. Catharsis is a dredging-up process. Many people don't really want to look very deeply into what exists below the surface of the ego. I have found that the work of catharsis creates more softness, sensitivity, and receptivity within me, while at the same time creating dynamic and healthy boundaries. When some barriers and armoring are broken down and released, softer aspects within myself are contacted. At the same time, some weaker part of myself receives acceptance and become more vital and powerful.

The question may come up as to why is it necessary to separate physically to deal with emotions. One of the telltale traits of emotion is that it enjoys discussion and argument, each one trying to convince the other why *he* or *she* is right. Emotion is full of ego. If you do stay in each other's presence when emotionally activated, it is really best if you can say "I feel . . ." and *only* talk about yourself. This is the most direct way to step out of emotion: to talk about what you are feeling at a deeper level, to express and release your hidden feelings. Bring the congestion of emotions from the solar plexus—where it is likely to have formed a knot—up to the heart, and get into your inner feelings for real. Do not make your partner responsible for creating unhappiness in you. Reach behind the emotion and find what is truly happening inside of you, the old hurts buried away that have nothing to do with this individual in front of you. He has only been a trigger for the cache of unexpressed feelings within.

Even if perhaps this person *is* in some way responsible for some of the hurts you carry from the past, the fact that you did not express your deeper feelings at that time, and repressed them instead, is really the issue in the present. If feelings had been authentically released at the time, they would not keep bubbling up inside of you. At least you would have felt a great deal better for having expressed the feelings, even if a particular issue remains unresolved between you. Through expression you cease to drag emotions around with you that accumulate year by year. Instead you keep yourself free from the past, straight and up to date.

Emotions are really toxins (which is what you feel swirling around in the fascia) that will poison the atmosphere, striking deadly blows at the person we most love, the one closest to us. This is a big problem—we unconsciously put all our unresolved feelings onto the person we most love, and thereby contaminate the love. We say the most awful things to our partner in an attempt to unburden ourselves of our emotions. Emotional statements stick like glue in the mind, and turn around in the thoughts endlessly, long after the fight is over. Did he *really* mean that? Am I really like *that?* And then *the mind will create more emotions from thinking over the past too much.* In truth, love cannot withstand too much emotion; it is like a delicate and fragile flower that requires awareness to keep it flourishing. Love will slowly slip through our fingers when we let emotion have the upper hand.

Conventional Sex Creates Emotionality

Another source of emotionality lies hidden in conventional sex. When energy moves downward, as it does in conventional sex with its conventional discharge, tension and anxiety are by-products.[1] This is why arguments and dissatisfactions easily follow. Sexual tensions eventually create an overcharge in woman, a subtle false-positive charge, and these accumulating tensions have to be discharged in some fashion. More often than not this happens through some kind of fighting, and often the tensions show up in premenstrual syndromes. When emotions are in the air they easily spawn excitement, which gives rise to the famous fucking-after-a-fight syndrome, a strategy commonly used to heal a rift between lovers. In reality, trying to patch up things like this is a vicious cycle, because through that same fuck women acquire more charge, which can flare up into emotion at any moment. This explains why, even in the absence of an argument, after a so-called good fuck a fight can start so easily.

Because of our emotional patterns, as women we can tend to get a bit high on emotions and begin to believe that this intensity is a part of love, that a good throwing around of china is an expression of our love. I have heard Barry Long say in a public gathering that all anger is, in reality, the result of sexual frustration. This certainly gives food for thought—and if you look at all the wars around us, and how little satisfying sex is being enjoyed on Earth, it appears that he speaks the truth. Women have diffi-culties and frustrations with conventional orgasm, so they are quite likely to have anger about this lurking within. Many women feel deep rage toward men for their abusive behavior, a rage that extends beyond the personal to the collective level.

Expressing Feelings in the Here and Now

In addition to (a) attempting to keep the past in the past by recognizing when emotion steps in, and (b) experimenting with relaxing into sex to avoid adding emotions to the store you already have, the art now becomes one of (c) staying in touch with your feelings, beginning to *feel what you are feeling*. To keep love fresh and free of emotion, it is essential to express feelings *as* they arise! Do not hang on to your feelings for an instant, unless you are in a hopelessly inappropriate situation. Move with the rising feeling and don't let your mind talk you out of it. Allow the tears to flow, the laughter to erupt, the roar to express itself, jump up and down, *do* something fast! Above all, do not repress feelings and in so doing form fresh emotions, which happens very quickly. Equally as quickly, any sadness, pain, anger, or frustration, if *fully* lived *as it is happening,* will have a life span of about eight seconds or so in intensity, after which it is all over.

When you practice consciously expressing anger there are a few hard and fast rules that come with it, and these are not to be broken under *any* circumstances. If you feel anger, do *not* direct it onto your partner, even if on the surface your emotions are convincing you that he is at fault. Do not touch him or do anything physically to hurt him—do not even face him. Turn to face in the opposite direction, showing him your back; then let a deep roar emerge from your belly.

The first time I allowed my anger to flow it was an unforgettable experience. In the very instant that I felt the rising anger for being blamed for something I did not do, I contacted a deep, roaring sound in my belly, that was so powerful it shot me up into the air to virtually touch the ceiling (which was higher than most ceilings are). By the time gravity pulled me back to terra firma a second or two later, it was all over. I felt no anger, no emotion, no resentment—nothing. I stepped back into the moment without hesitation, ready and willing to continue communicating.

When anger arises, welcome it knowing that it is an old tension existing within you and it can be transformed. By expressing it for yourself you are released from its restrictive grip. Contacting feelings is a cleansing experience—energy that was locked suddenly becomes available. When you express a feeling or transform an emotion you feel lighter, expanded and fresh, connected to your partner, open and soft, clear and radiant, even loving. Emotions bring the experience of quite opposite qualities: darkness and gloom, despair and collapse. The whole range of positive experiences is what shows up when you share your feelings.

Woman Needs to Make Love for Her Continuing Health

Just as tension is the by-product of energy moving downward (as in conventional sex), silence is the outcome of energy moving upward (as in tantric sex or meditation).[2] Relaxing into sex brings you into a state of being that is quite apart from the whole range of emotions. Through relaxing and reaching the orgasmic state, we reach a rare peace and fulfillment, a state in which our energy is regenerated and we become filled with love, not only for the beloved but for any person around us. As energy moves upward through the centers (chakras) it cleanses them, purifies them, and makes them dynamic and alive.

However, at present women suffer extreme menstrual syndromes with hormonal ups and downs and lack of self-value alongside fears of aging, menopausal anxieties, and disappointment and often disinterest in sex. At a certain point sex is considered by many women to be too much hard work with very little reward, and for this reason they give it up. I heard a research statistic mentioned by a U.S. television show host recently revealing that 45 percent of happily married couples did not have sex in the last six months!

For men, too, the situation is dire. Until given the chance to enjoy the flowering of sex through direct experience, man cannot imagine it. And since excitement and ejaculation are the only tricks he knows, he is not giving much thought to trying something different. These tricks, however, are only superficially satisfying, while in the depths a bubbling sexual pool remains untapped. A man's inability to channel his real life force leads to frustration, aggression, anger, restlessness, obsessive fantasizing about sex—in sex and out of sex—and all manner of sexual perversions. When the tantric energy circulates freely through him he feels himself, finally, as more of a man. At the end of a workshop recently I overheard a man saying to Raja, my partner, "This is the first time in my life of fifty-four years that I have been given any insights or guidance on what it means to be a man." And that was not the first time I've heard this.

When a woman knows it is possible to use her sexual energy rightfully, allowing it to circulate throughout the body orgasmically, her sense of self changes and she *wants* to make love. Sex becomes less to do with the other or with getting something and becomes more a way of valuing and loving oneself, of being with oneself. With insight into her body mechanisms she is able to direct her sexual energy and so be more in command of her life. The process of the body getting older and perhaps less attractive becomes of no real concern, in the sense that she knows how to attract the male principle when a man is in her presence, how to draw and drink from him, through understanding the deeper layers of sexual energy. It has nothing to do with how she looks or how old she is. She bypasses the superficiality of sex and steps directly into the female element, which is passive, relaxed, receptive, sweet, serene, open. Such an ambience in itself stimulates man to respond to woman in a way quite different from how he usually responds.

Perhaps only a woman can really and truly break the cycle of unconsciousness in sex. When sex is balanced and in accord with her female design, a woman has some leverage, some authority in sex, and a new confidence in herself. Her man will be in wonder and even a bit awestruck to learn how the same elements—the penis and the vagina—can produce two such vastly different experiences.

The Emotion of Jealousy

Jealousy is perhaps the most debilitating and excruciating of emotions, more frequently experienced by women than by men. Jealousy is concerned with possessing and controlling another person; it is not an expression of love for that person. Jealousy has its roots in comparison, and we are taught to compare ourselves in all kinds of ways, particularly in the sexual sphere. Easily and instantly we can have overwhelming feelings of inadequacy and feel threatened by another woman giving or receiving attentions from the man we love. In the conventional picture, a new and fresh pretty, tilted face represents a bit of excitement to a man, excitement being his main stimulus for sex at present. However, when a woman steps away from excitement as the basis of the sexual experience, she finds a real rootedness in her deeper self; then she is not so easily knocked off center.

Comparison is a useless activity because each individual is unique and incomparable, and once this understanding settles in you, it is possible for jealousy to disappear. Sex certainly creates jealousy, but jealousy is a secondary thing. So it is not a question of how to drop jealousy. Jealousy cannot easily be dropped while we are trapped in conventional sex. The question therefore is how to transform sex into love. And in this love, jealousy disappears.

Don't repress it, express it. Sit in your room, close the doors, bring your jealousy into focus. Watch it, see it, let it take as strong a flame as possible. Let it become a strong flame, burn into it and see what it is. And don't from the very beginning say that this is ugly, because that very idea that this is ugly will repress the jealousy, will not allow it total expression. No opinions. Just try to see the existential effect of what jealousy is, the existential fact. No interpretations, no ideologies. Just let the jealousy be there. Look into it, look deeply into it and so do with anger, so do with sadness, hatred, possessiveness. And by and by you will see that just by seeing through things you start getting a transcendental feeling that you are just a witness; the identity is broken. The identity is broken only when you encounter something within you.

OSHO, TRANSCRIBED TEACHINGS,

TAO: THE PATHLESS PATH

Divesting Interest in Peak Orgasm and Ejaculation

We know that many a man is obsessed with producing a peak orgasm for a woman because it validates him as a lover. And we understand that this attitude has grave consequences, for both men and women—that peak orgasms leave a residue of tension that become a source of emotions in woman (and man), and that, in trying to produce excitement and orgasm in woman, man easily ejaculates, which is against a woman's long-term interests.

But some women are equally identified with their lover's ejaculation. They say quite clearly that, for them, their man's orgasm is an essential part of the sexual act. A woman of this persuasion feels that in the very moment of releasing his semen he gives himself utterly to her, he shares something of his essence that he can do with no one else. In reality, each ejaculation is an enormous disempowerment of man, for it represents an incalculable amount of energy in sperm life—approximately two hundred *million* to five hundred *million* sperms, or potential human beings, per ejaculation. Huge amounts of creativity are lost by the male species through habitual and uncontrollable ejaculation! Ejaculation has become the norm, and woman can easily get into supporting man in this.

Yet with her capacity to influence the sex act by discovering the source of her orgasm in her breasts, any woman can begin reconfiguring her sexual reality to guarantee a life of love and a love free of emotion. The fragrance of a woman settled in her essence exerts an attractive force on man that alters the whole nature of the sexual act—it is a dimensional shift.

The stakes are enormous. Until a woman approaches sexuality in a truly feminine manner it is difficult or impossible for a man to change. Until man can manage to satisfy one woman utterly and completely, he will never feel himself to be a true man, in spite of any other achievements and successes. The need for man to feel himself as masculine, for woman to feel herself as feminine, and for both to have orgasmic experiences through each other is a burning need for humanity today. Without this spiritual sexual expression the human race will slowly die from starvation and become extinct through a dire shortage of love.

The Division between Sex and Heart's Love

Perhaps most women have at times (if not all the time) experienced a drastic and dramatic split between the experience of sex and the feelings of love. Sex can so easily feel dirty and animal and uncaring while love is something sweet and pure and beautiful. A majority of women have had countless experiences of loveless sex, and as a result many women choose a sexless life, at the same time attempting to love a man very dearly. Or instead, they choose to be alone.

But this solution of abandoning sex because it is not deeply moving comes at some cost to woman herself. As mentioned, lack of love and loving in woman results in all kinds of ill health, psychological disturbances, and emotional problems. For a woman, sex itself is not a dire need while love is an absolute need, and always remains one to the end of her life. The effort lies in bringing these two seemingly conflicting worlds into synchronicity. The route to that state is to connect sex with the heart (and love) *through* sex, not by avoiding it. Sex with any level of awareness creates love naturally, as a by-product; it follows simply and sweetly. Awareness is alchemical. Combining these two poles in her own body— sex and love, the earthly and the otherworldly—is the optimum for health and continued happiness for women.

Many women report that sometimes the heart feels like it is being touched internally, penetrated and opened by the penis, particularly when the penetration is deep and prolonged as suggested in chapter 6. When physical love reaches to this level of exchange through polarity, love is generated as a tangible reality between a man and a woman. In being so profoundly touched, woman connects with her love and in overflow showers love on man, thereby completing the circuit of love and joy. Remember this again and again: *any* level of awareness in sex will create love—it is the awareness itself that transforms sex into love. To repeat a common phrase: it is not what we do but how we do it. Woman is love, this is the quintessence of her very soul; thus, to her love is as essential as food. She requires the opportunity to relax into her feminine nature and receive the contentment and regeneration of orgasmic experiences to sustain her life. The sincerity and willingness of a man is clearly a contributing factor to woman's orgasmic experiences, but the responsibility—even for this—lies in woman's hands. Through sex woman can regain her original power as female.

One Woman's Journey

I am fortunate to be able to include here a written report by a woman from Switzerland, now a good friend, whom I first met during a "Making Love" retreat several years ago. She and her partner have been experimenting very sincerely with tantra since then. Recently I slipped her an email asking her to write, if she wished, a few lines to quickly encapsulate her experience. Instead of the two or three lines I expected she sent a comprehensive and sincere assessment of her transformation, and I am grateful to her for doing so. Her experience can be an encouragement and inspiration to every woman.

The most amazing development in our sexuality and lovemaking is this: The plugging in (the "tantric quickie"), which we do at least twice a day when we are together [they live together half of the week] is somehow healing deep wounds in our bodies *and* souls without our conscious effort or contribution. Fully beyond our heads (quite unusual for us), the bodies are doing this healing all by themselves! I enjoy sex much more, am always ready to make love provided there is enough time, and the pressure to perform is gone, as well as the fear of being hurt again. S. now knows his penis can come into my vagina anytime, which makes it less desirable somehow. But also, his urgent physical "baby needs" are finally fulfilled. He really seems to finally get what he needed most throughout his life with the plugging in!

So when we are exhausted from working too much, we now peacefully plug in and go to sleep instead of the earlier dramas of having to have an exciting sex act at any cost because if we didn't have sex every day, something wasn't normal in the relationship (thus spending two or more difficult hours trying to achieve something, under performance pressure, with fancy underwear and toys, etc., instead of sleeping, which was what our bodies really needed . . .). When we wake up at night, we either plug in again or make love. The first one to awaken in the morning asks the other one to plug in once more.

This has made us into peaceful human beings—no more fighting in the office, which we did daily before we learned from you. And if we do fight, we know that we are not taking enough time for love and have skipped our weekly appointments for making love. This skipping unfortunately still happens quite often. We are so performance-driven and responsible for our company, with twelve employees, and our garden, that we have difficulties with making time for love a top priority. (Interestingly, when we do just that and go away for a full week to a "Making Love" workshop, orders come in like crazy—this has happened two times now!) S. is getting what he needs to a point where I feel he really wants me as his partner, and has stopped wondering if there is anyone better out there. I feel the same way, especially when life with him is not stressful. Then it's all that I have ever dreamed of; we come into love deeper and deeper! We're even talking about getting married.

The other great help was your teaching about the difference between emotions and feelings. We are still both working hard at the "daring to express our feelings" part. I still sometimes don't dare to express them in order to minimize stress when it is already here. But then my resentments toward the stress come out in other ways, in aggressions—so I don't serve the whole if I don't say what I feel! My head knows that, but the little girl inside is still afraid to lose the love she needs so badly.

I'm working on that. It was amazing how few times we had to go jogging or screaming or cleaning before we recognized being emotional quickly enough to stop the fighting. Only a total of about five times— but we are used to recognizing patterns amongst the two of us, which was also very helpful. My breasts are still very sensitive and accept touch only when it happens in a fully loving way. They want S.'s or my own hands to go away immediately again when they feel manipulated. This is a tough one. It would take several sessions of loving touch to more easily welcome touch at my breasts—I better start planning for them!

In our third time of attending your "Making Love" workshop I had a beautiful release inside. A great pain came up in my vagina or uterus shortly before my period. I usually never have that. When I got up at night to go to the toilet and came back, it had gotten so bad I woke up S. and asked him to plug in to make it better. We started talking about the pain, and at some point I said "I carry this pain with pride." S. asked "For whom?" and I instantly replied "For my father, of course." S. said, "But your father doesn't see you, is not interested in you, and thinks you're crazy anyway!" All of which is true. I realized the little girl in me still does everything she can to win her father's love, because she wasn't able to reach him with her great love for him when she was little. So I took my pillow (standing for the little girl) into my arms and finally cried about this. The tears and mourning washed away my core belief that love doesn't have a chance (because it didn't have one back then). This belief had led to my subtle dismantling of love whenever it showed itself, with a little criticism here and some aggression there—I seem to have done that in order not to reexperience the disappointment of not reaching somebody with my love, which was so overwhelmingly big when I was a child and had left me so very lonely. After the crying and recognizing what it was telling me, the pain in my belly slowly went away. I'm very careful now to give love a real chance, especially with S. and my children. . . .

Women Sharing Experiences

"Another 'aha!' realization that keeps coming to me is never to take anything of my partner's response as personal *and* not to exclude anything. It reminds me of the well-used phrase 'Tantra does not exclude anything.' I also had to let go very early in the process of this idea and identification that I am a very fucked up and wounded woman. To disengage from the emotional, over and over, is a delight."

"I connected with my own rejection wound. I've been in it for days—in pain and panic and not able to see my way. It's like a rewinding. Right now I'm back to ages seven to eleven, realizing how much this little flower has been abused. I feel compassion for myself, my partner, all the unconsciousness. . . . From this wound I have rejected others, especially men. Everything has been about projection. I cried for hours."

"The wounds seem all to be in the heart—all about receiving love and giving love. When a lot of rejection is there, there is a closing to receiving love and a disbelief that my love has value to a man."

"Today I really connected with the eyes as a key. Keeping eye contact kept us both present and lifted me right out of the emotions and past movies, and I found that I can trust my intuition about how to move into this space. Also, opening my eyes with the focus being 'in' and not 'out' helps me to stay connected almost as much as if I have my eyes closed."

"I had major energy release happening during the lovemaking; it was electrical. The non-movement brought up all my 'no' to penetration, 'no' to man."

"After six or seven days I felt so much energy building up inside. We had an exquisite meeting where I felt all the boundaries in my vagina melt away, which made my man's erection very strong. We were very blissful, present for a long time. After that for three days everything went the other way, my Christian judgments coming in full force—bad sleep, feeling restless and prudish, all kind of things came up for me. Our sexual meetings have gone to a deeper level it seems. The mind freaks out, reacts; the vagina has become more and more tense to a point that the whole pelvic floor is in contraction. This morning it was impossible to make love. We talked through our genitals—abuse was strong on both sides—both from outside. I have three rapes in my history as well as my personal abuse of my genitals by fucking when I didn't feel like it. It is still tight everywhere, but strangely enough, by sharing our tightness, lying very close together, I still feel very connected to my partner and loving and friendly."

"I got the impression I never learned so much about real love as I did in this week. I was always looking for this feeling and hoping I would meet it one day. Yes, I came near to it but in a different way in certain moments in meditations in the awareness training I've done over the past ten years. But in my daily life with my husband I had many returning moments of sadness. Our relationship was really good and deep; we have been together for twenty-three years and I always had the impression we loved each other, were there for each other, cared about the other, went through difficult times together, enjoyed life together, had good conventional sex, all was so good, and—there was a big and—I many times felt a big sadness deep in me. I had this 'idea' of love that I felt was covered over on a very deep level. In all these years I carried big doubts within myself. Doubts about whether I really loved my man compared to the love I had as an 'idea.' Then I doubted whether that love could exist on our Earth-level of existence. I carried all these questions in me. During the week I started to get closer to real love. I could not imagine that my love for my man could get so strong and fine at the same time. We spent such wonderful hours, we shared so many things, I was crying sometimes just because I was so happy to get closer to this deep love. I am so thankful for this big gift!"

Tantric Inspiration

This has been my observation: It is difficult for people to love, but there is one thing that is even more difficult than to love, and that is to receive love. To love is difficult, but to receive love is almost impossible. Why? Because to love is in a way simple, and one can do it because it is not against the ego. When you love somebody you are giving something, and the ego feels enhanced. You have the upper hand, you are the giver, and the other is at the receiving end. You feel very good; your ego feels enhanced, puffed up. But when you receive love, you can't have the upper hand. Receiving, your ego feels hurt. Receiving love is more difficult than giving love. And one has to learn both—to give and receive.

And to receive is going to transform you more than giving can do, because in receiving love your ego starts disappearing.

OSHO, TRANSCRIBED TEACHINGS,
I SAY UNTO YOU, (VOL. 1)

Question on Emotions

[This passage begins with a personal question by a female disciple to Osho.]

Beloved Master,

So often a feeling that I can't describe fills my heart and my whole being. During the other morning's discourse it felt like overwhelming love for you and the whole. But now I realize that the same feeling or a very, very similar feeling also comes up in fear, anguish, throbbing pain, helplessness, and frustration. I am trembling and confused. Beloved Master, can you say something?

Osho answers:

There is certainly something very similar in very different emotions: the overwhelmingness. It may be love, it may be hate, it may be anger—it can be anything. If it is too much then it gives you a sense of being over-whelmed by something. Even pain and suffering can create the same experience, but overwhelmingness has no value in itself. It simply shows you are an emotional being.

This is typically the indication of an emotional personality. When it is anger, it is all anger. And when it is love, it is all love. It almost becomes drunk with the emotion, blind. And whatever action comes out of it is wrong. Even if it is overwhelming love, the action that will come out of it is not going to be right.

Reduced to its base, whenever you are overwhelmed by any emotion you lose all reason, you lose all sensitivity, you lose your heart in it. It becomes almost like a dark cloud in which you are lost. Then whatever you do is going to be wrong.

Love is not to be a part of your emotions. Ordinarily that's what people think and experience, but anything overwhelming is very unstable. It comes like a wind and passes by, leaving you behind, empty, shattered, in sadness and in sorrow.

According to those who know man's whole being—his mind, his heart, and his being—love has to be an expression of your being, not an emotion. Emotion is very fragile, very changing. One moment it seems that is all. Another moment you are simply empty.

So the first thing to do is take love out of this crowd of overwhelming emotions. Love is not overwhelming. On the contrary, love is a tremendous insight, clarity, sensitivity, awareness. But that kind of love rarely exists, because very few people ever reach to their being.

OSHO, TRANSCRIBED TEACHINGS,
OM SHANTIH SHANTIH SHANTIH

Awareness and Sensitivity Exercise
Self-Massage of the Solar Plexus

If you find the solar plexus congested or uncomfortable at any time, it is very important to dissolve the tensions that have collected there; otherwise you may discharge them in other ways. Massage is helpful for increasing awareness of the area.

Lie on your back with your arms at your sides, in an aligned position as suggested in previous exercises, with about twenty to thirty minutes to yourself. Take a few deep breaths into the belly and solar plexus area. Then make your fingertips into a pointy tool by placing them back to back, with fingernails touching. Bring your hands to the solar plexus area and very lightly place this tool on the skin about half way between the arch of your rib cage and your navel. Rest here for a few moments using hardly any pressure—like a butterfly alighting on a flower—and soon you will begin to feel the heartbeat pulsing in the solar plexus. If you feel no pulse after several minutes, increase the pressure slightly. Keep your attention on your fingertips and feel the pulsing of the heart.

After a few minutes pull the fingers away from the heartbeat but don't lose contact with the skin. It is a fraction of a movement, just a hairbreadth. Take two or three nice deep breaths through the solar plexus into the belly, and then deepen your contact again to return your fingertips to the pulse of the heartbeat. Continue this process of feeling the pulse and then giving the pulse space by pulling away for as long as you are comfortable with the exercise. When you have finished, pull away from the solar plexus extremely slowly. Place one hand on top of the other over the solar plexus, keeping your eyes closed and resting for a few minutes.

Awareness and Sensitivity Exercise
Cathartic Exercise for Repressed Emotions

It is an excellent idea to create the space to intentionally contact unexpressed anger. Whenever you feel that you cannot get below the stomach, that you are not reaching into your belly, when you feel somehow superficial, you can walk and pant like a dog. You will need three things: a half hour of privacy; a room with the door closed; and, ideally, the liberty to make some sound without arousing the curiosity of your neighbors. This kind of anger is usually embedded deep in the body, which makes it difficult to work with directly. However, indirectly something can be done with anger so as to release accumulated frustrations.

Simply pretend that you are a dog by letting your tongue stick out and hang down. Walk around on the floor on all fours (hands and knees) and take fast panting breaths through your mouth. As you do this, the passage down the throat to the belly will open. Pant for thirty minutes and soon anger will flow easily and beautifully. Let your whole body become involved in it. You can even bark and growl at your reflection in the mirror.

If anger is a constant stumbling block for you, I suggest you do this panting exercise daily for a period of about three weeks. Once anger is released, you will have the feeling of body energies awakened very deeply and you will feel an inner freedom—you will no longer be in bondage to unexpressed feelings held in the body.

11

Woman as Lover During Menstruation, Fertility, Pregnancy, Motherhood, and Menopause

A woman, simply by virtue of being a woman with the capacity to bear children, is subject to the influence of hormones that affect her life and her sexual expression in powerful ways, and these must not be underestimated. A whole class of these effects is produced by the very knowledge that, for much of her life, sex for a woman is inextricably linked with the possibility of pregnancy. It starts with menstruation at puberty, and from then onward in many cases an unadulterated fear of accidentally getting pregnant lies between a woman and her full immersion into sex. Deep-seated fear can be a great hindrance to the experience of sex as something natural and beautiful.

The Contraception Issue

Many women, particularly in their teenage years, are bound to have had experiences of an excruciating longing to have sex and a simultaneously profound *no* to it. Usually in these circumstances the contraception issue has not been addressed or acted upon. This inner conflict of yes/no creates great tension in a woman and affects her ability to genuinely open up, to herself and to a man. And even if she does open up, she is likely to retain a subtle *no* of underlying resistance, when so much is at stake. If a woman is compelled to set out with a basic unwillingness to open up and relax, this contraction does not help the expansion of female energy. Tensions about pregnancy will influence and affect a woman's presence, her pleasure, and her entire perception of sex.

Fertility awareness becomes essential if a woman really wants to let go into lovemaking. Without it, the riskiness of the situation, the resistance to it and the wanting of it, can serve to intensify the excitement to a point that she will willy-nilly thrust herself into the experience, throwing all caution to the wind. It starts out with a no, and yet the woman is slowly getting excited, still saying no but enjoying the sexual feelings. At a certain point the excitement reaches a peak with the overwhelming desire for penetration, and the *no* rapidly flips on its head into a *yes*, and this is certainly not the moment to halt the proceedings to insert a diaphragm or roll on a condom. Thrusting oneself into sex like this is to enter the act with an already high level of excitement, with less awareness, and usually with the desire for orgasm—all of which pretty much guarantees ejaculation. Which of course makes the risks of pregnancy even higher.

For all of these reasons it is really essential that a woman, especially when young, take complete responsibility for contraception and not leave it up to the man. A woman does herself a great service if she takes precautions against unwanted pregnancy: much energy is liberated into the sexual experience. A woman who has had the joy of a vasectomized man entering her life will know what an incredible relief it is not to even *think* about contraception. Not ever! Making love becomes so joyful and easy—just an unconditional *yes* away.

Often women in workshops will ask the question, "What about making love during menstruation—is it good or bad?" Basically, to make love at this time is perfectly fine; it is a super-safe time relative to the fertility cycle and can even ease menstrual symptoms such pain or irritability. It really depends on the personal choice and preferences of the two people involved. There are no general rules to be made and each woman has to find her own way with her partner in this.

When Sex and Fertility Make Friends

Keeping track of a woman's fertility cycle is the most helpful way to avoid or invite pregnancy. Perhaps the best tool for this is the Sympto-Thermal Method. Having a working knowledge of this method empowers women, in that they remain in closer contact to the cycles of their bodies and puts them in a position to have greater control over contraception. Nature gives us subtle signs telling us when a woman is fertile: ovulation is accompanied by a temperature rise (sympto-thermal), which indicates the passing of an egg being released from the ovaries to travel down the fallopian tubes to the womb. At the same time, there are changes in the cervical fluid. In the Sympto-Thermal Method, the temperature rise is always interpreted in correlation to cervical fluid observation, and together these reveal ovarian activity. This method is taught by two major world organizations: a Catholic organization called the Natural Family Planning (NFP) Institute and the non-religious-affiliated Fertility Awareness Method (FAM) schools. Instructions in the Sympto-Thermal Method can be obtained from these organizations and others all over the world. Some women manage to learn the method on their own just by reading a competent book, but it is recommended that they discuss their charts at least once with a Sympto-Thermal counselor and, importantly, that they fully include their partners.

It is commonly understood that having sex but refraining from ejaculation is not a sufficiently safe form of contraception. Accordingly, the Sympto-Thermal Method, the so-called "natural contraception" method, is not considered sufficiently safe by its antagonists. Instead, the multi-billion-dollar hormone industry, and thus, most gynecologists and other doctors, discourage women from getting involved with their own fertility cycles. Advocates of the natural approach insist that the Sympto-Thermal Method is the best-kept secret around, and the underlying reason is monetary: consumption of expensive pills to forget about body cycles is preferred, and so there is precious little promotion of self awareness and how to better take care of ourselves.

For women who do wish to know more about this method, I have included a detailed introduction in the appendix at the back of the book. Although you should not consider this account complete, I have included all the contact information you will need on how to learn more.

Choosing to Have a Child

When a woman feels ready to have a child and truly wishes for one, it is very much advantageous to all concerned to *consciously* conceive that child, to ensure that the pregnancy results from a planned ejaculation to coincide with ovulation, not an accidental ejaculation. A couple should build a special ritual around such a conception experience, creating a temple for making love, providing a sacred space into which to invite a new being into life. A child entering the world is easily able to sense welcome or a lack of welcome; she feels how she has been longed for or accommodated by the new parents, whether they have changed joyfully or adjusted reluctantly to fit her into their usually already busy lives. Feelings of being unwelcome will be in force in this new being in spite of all of the loving attentions that may subsequently be poured on her. A child who has truly been invited into the world displays a completely different psychology and life force.

One basic way in which a baby can sense the lack of welcome on planet Earth is through a lack of breast-feeding. Many mothers today do not have the time or the patience to devote themselves to breast-feeding, and further, some women fear they will ruin their breasts by breast-feeding and thereby decrease their sexual attractiveness. Breast milk contains all the vital ingredients essential for developing a healthy immune system in a child, so breast-feeding is basic to human life. Yet today not many women breast-feed their children for more than a few weeks. Much less common is breast-feeding for twelve to eighteen months.

Sex during Pregnancy

Pregnancy, planned or not, raises the question of how to proceed with a sexual life for the following nine months. As the pregnancy advances many women become reluctant to engage in sex, becoming concerned that in some way the baby will be hurt through sex, and this concern increases as the pregnancy progresses. This is perhaps the first time that a woman becomes conscious of the aggressive, unloving quality of the conventional sexual exchange. Feeling a need to protect her unborn child, she begins to turn away from sexual overtures by her man. This withdrawal often creates tensions within the relationship; by the time the baby arrives, not much sex has been had at all in the preceding months.

With the conscious and loving tantric approach to sex, and soft penetration with the possibility of erection in the vagina as described in chapter 8, sex is easy to engage in. It is such a completely organic approach that a woman will feel in herself that absolutely no harm can come to the fetus. On the contrary, women in my workshops who have attended in the seventh to the ninth month of pregnancy all report a positive response from the fetus. Tantric sex creates more space for the baby, because the belly relaxes. The movement of the fetus increases, and in some cases tantric lovemaking has even stimulated the act of the fetus turning to the head-down position important for birth. The life force generated during sex radiates through the whole body, with beneficial outcome for both mother and child. It can act as a preparation for birth. In addition, this lovemaking nourishes the loving bond between man and woman, which is the foundation of parenthood.

Sex after Birth and while Breast-feeding

After the birth of a child, a woman's reluctance to engage in sex tends to increase. Some of this disinclination can be an outcome of the birth experience itself and the intensely physical process a woman goes through. If it was a difficult birth, with tears and stitches at the entrance of the vagina for instance, a woman will feel naturally unwilling to open up to sex. A tantric friend of mine reported that she had two completely opposite experiences giving birth: the first was very hard and very long and the second took only six hours. Though the second birth was intense, it was a natural birth and was a very empowering experience. After the birth of her first child she noticed she could not even entertain the *thought* of getting interested "down there"—it seemed that feeling sexual was simply light years away. My friend required five months of healing before she felt physically available to make love with her husband. When she finally agreed, she experienced the soft penetration and presence of the penis inside her as a tremendously healing experience. Many tears and tensions were able to flow out of her system. In contrast, with her second child she resumed lovemaking (tantric style, as she had done up to the birth) shortly after the birth and continues to make love regularly (one to four times a week), along with breast-feeding and caring for her two children.

In the case of cesarean birth there is often pain and discomfort associated with the surgery and healing of the wound, as well as a general sensation of being cut off from the pelvic basin—the genitals and pelvic floor. With vaginal birth, many women are given an episiotomy—a cut from the vaginal entrance into the perineum—as a routine procedure that is done with the intention of preventing the possibility of any tearing during birth. In these cases penetration is associated with pain in the vagina. So it follows that if birth has occurred without surgical invasion or difficulties, the mother is more likely to be open to sexual exchange. Her body is relatively intact and carrying no traumas that need time to heal in the body and the psyche.

Apparent Loss of Libido after Birth

As a creative expression of the female element, giving birth is a profoundly transforming process for a woman. For some women the birth process can be an orgasmic experience. Birth energetically expands a woman's system and thereby increases her overall receptivity and sensitivity. As a consequence of giving birth a woman feels more feminine, more connected to her innate female nature.

So it is quite understandable that, in these new circumstances, a new mother is not as interested in sex as she was before the birth—in sex of the conventional kind, at any rate, in which her delicate feminine senses are transgressed. The conscious, tantric approach to sex poses no problems for a woman because it does not involve the machinations and strenuousness demanded by convention. Perhaps the commonly experienced loss of libido after childbirth is due to nothing other than resistance to the conventional approach to sex—not a resistance to sex itself. For a woman as mother, it is important to move into the spiritual expression of sex, which requires raising that same energy that produced the child. This will bring her, as woman, more love, vitality, and wisdom. Sex is a powerful way of indirectly nourishing a child.

At present in the field of medicine the loss of libido is attributed to prolactin, a hormone that is secreted after giving birth and is absolutely necessary for breast-feeding. Prolactin is a physiological requirement of the body, because without it the breast milk is unable flow. Prolactin works as a relaxant for the breasts, and naturally calms and relaxes the mother in preparation for breast-feeding. Incidentally, prolactin is also used in psychiatry for its calming effects. Knowing the role of prolactin in milk production, a woman can feel more relaxed about the calm state of her libido. It is an internal body process, so to feel tired or lacking energy while breast-feeding a child is perfectly normal. As well, breast-feeding represents a huge commitment, as an adequate schedule is about six or seven times a day for at least four to six months. So when a woman does not feel attracted to the rigors of normal sex, it may be unrealistic to call it a loss of libido!

Breast-Feeding Enhances Lovemaking

In the tantric picture, to be relaxed is actually considered a great advantage, and a woman will be naturally more open and receptive while she is breast-feeding—a gift! (Soft penetration is quite feasible during breast-feeding itself.) It is possible also to support the flow from the breasts by connecting with the inner energy circle flowing from the breasts to the vagina and back again to the breasts. A tantric friend of mine who breast-feeds with awareness of the breasts as the positive downward-radiating pole says she finds the experience very nourishing; it even gives her a certain sexual fulfillment by virtue of completing her inner circle. She says that the circular connection, the tuning in to her body, creates a calm, peaceful atmosphere around her, which gives the baby a sense of security, and this in turn helps the baby relax into drinking. By making the experience a nourishing one for herself, a woman can avoid exhaustion or irritability, extreme sensitivity in the nipples, and feeling empty and drained of reserves after feeding.

Remember, breast-feeding prevents ovulation, so as long as a woman is breast-feeding she is protected by natural contraception.* You can add this to the advantages of breast-feeding. It is really the perfect period of time for making love. You can be almost certain that during this time there will be no ovulation, which gives you time to get back in sync with your partner. A woman can be infertile for about eighteen months if she breast-feeds for this length of time; however, after six months she should seek more information from a fertility counselor.

The World Health Organization recommends a minimum of one year of breast-feeding, which makes it difficult or impossible for a new mother to work away from the home. In Sweden, mothers are paid by the government for one year to assist them financially in order to encourage breast-feeding, in recognition of the vital importance of mother's milk to the building of a child's immune system and future health.

All in all, sex after giving birth can be a great healing force, and women are encouraged not to abandon being a lover when becoming a mother. In the tantric context one starts to view life very differently, to see that a conscious approach in sex can be a unifying force, as things that are normally held apart (sex and parenthood) are brought together in harmony. You can engage in unassertive tantric sex in the vicinity of babies because it is a loving and natural happening—unlike conventional sex, which is more animalistic and places adults in an embarrassing situation when children happen in on them.

---

*The contraceptive protection is about 95 percent as long as a woman is breast-feeding her baby at least six times a day; not more than six hours pass between feedings; and the baby is consuming no other liquids in addition to the breast milk. If these rules are not followed, ovulation could occur.

Sex and Parenthood

Over and above the actual birth experience and its impact on a woman's sexual willingness, birth marks the significant transition from woman to mother. It is an experience of great energy expansion; with it a woman's energy changes and becomes more feminine, receptive, and loving. The qualities of motherhood are instilled through the birth process. A total shift in consciousness occurs—love wells up from an inner source and flowers into an utter devotion to the well-being of this fragile new life. Woman becomes 100 percent present to the needs of her child. A natural absorption with the child makes her less accessible to man, and it may become impossible to tear herself away from tending to the baby to notice the needs of her partner. From a woman's perspective it can seem an insurmountable effort at this time to open up to making love and to her man himself.

However, the love between a couple really needs to be nourished. Lavishing attentions on the child and excluding the man leads to the possibility of the man feeling unwanted, getting restless, and seeking "entertainment" elsewhere. It is well documented that, when a man is continually refused sex by his woman-turned-mother in the early years of parenthood, his eyes will start to roam. When sex is not available at home, inevitably he will find alternative sources. Thus it happens frequently that a man will move on permanently to greener pastures, leaving a woman stranded, babe and all.

Given the innate male-female polarities, sex is more essential for the male; it is not as optional as it is for women. As passive pole, women do not really appreciate this important difference between the sexes. I remember a twenty-year-old mother recently telling me, with innocent girlish surprise on her face, that she had *no* idea that sex was so important to a man. This sharing followed a spate of arguments with her man over the issue of availability for sex, which had some frightening emotional touches to it.

Well, the simple truth is that sex is extremely important for a man. A mother must find a balance between the two, and understand that love between man and woman will sustain the love for the child and the harmony in the home.

A new mother is often overconcerned about a child's physical needs and comfort, smothering the baby with attention instead of attending to the ambience surrounding the baby. As *mother* a woman has responsibility to her child and as *woman* she has responsibility to her man, the father of her child—an almost equal responsibility, if she wants her child to grow up in the ambience of love rather than conflict. And this is not to mention the responsibility of woman to *herself* to obtain nourishment and love and tenderness and so avoid the buildup of emotions. The love field that bonds and surrounds the parents is as vital a food to a young child as is the breast milk of the mother. Children are extremely sensitive to this; they draw on the nourishment love provides, and where there is an absence of harmony and lack of love there is a shrinking (due to fear) in the core of the child's energy system. They become tense and wary, possibly restless and demanding, even if well fed and properly taken care of. If this unlovingness continues and the years accumulate, the children will grow up to be overly emotional and afraid and not as filled with love as they might otherwise have been.

Parents are not aware of this when they fight in front of their children. When a sensitive new life is engulfed by tensions and arguments, a defensive, contracting fear sets in and a child easily grows up learning to express herself with an emotional personality; thus problems in life and relating begin. Parents need to keep all evidence of their fights away from their children. They need to take responsibility for their states of emotionality, following the steps suggested in chapter 10, to prevent the toxic vibrations of emotionality from having an influence on a child. Children are exceptionally sensitive to the atmosphere between the parents for as long as they are living at home, which can be for seventeen years or more. Many parents have said that when they started to make love more often, after participating in my workshop, it had a positive impact on the children. The children became less demanding and more content in themselves, and the usual squabbles between the children diminished dramatically. Parents concern themselves with informing and educating their children in any number of ways, yet they often overlook the basic requirement of love in a family, the very glue that keeps a family together. Parents who make love and live a loving life as a consequence give the best possible preparation and education to their children.

Sex during and after Menopause

The final cycle through which all women pass, whether they have had a child or not, is menopause—the ceasing of monthly menstrual bleeding. Many women hold menstruation dear, as it represents their womanhood. Thus many a woman begins to dread menopause because it appears as a threat to her femininity and attractiveness.

But this is true only when you look through conventional eyes. If a woman makes an attempt to step away from conditioned sex (with luck, early in her life, though it really is never too late to start), she receives a profound understanding of femininity and the real nature of sexual attraction. She knows it has nothing to do with outer appearance but with an ageless and powerful force residing within her. This brings a confidence and clarity way beyond the limiting concerns of the physical aging process. In fact, as you embrace tantric sex more and more, you feel better and better about yourself and getting older holds no great anxiety. Of course, the body itself may manifest a few telling signs, but the spirit remains ever young. A woman who learns the art of tantra empowers herself to make love until the end of her days, if this is her wish, without need to give it up with menopause and then old age.

Many women report that penetration becomes extremely painful during menopause, and I have met women in workshops in a relationship crisis because of this. Some have been unable to have sex for several years because of this uncomfortable symptom. Adding to this problem can be a lack of lubrication often experienced during this phase of hormonal change. Conventional sex becomes impossible for many women during menopause. However, tantra offers us the possibility of soft penetration, from which an erection is able to grow, and women who have tried this say there is absolutely no pain. Suddenly new doors open through which lovemaking can enter again in all its glory.

In my experience of working with women in menopause I can report that a conscious approach in sex is of great benefit. Women who have commenced with a tantric approach during menopause say they very definitely notice a relaxation of many of the menopausal symptoms. Hot flashes, for example, flow down to the ground as if a channel has been opened. Some of the emotional difficulties are also relieved. Unfortunately there is not enough research being done in this area; however, a body of evidence is bound to emerge as more and more women begin to embrace tantric principles.

Menopause marks the time of a great rise in creativity for a woman— now free from the bondage of her hormonal aspect (the biological expression of sex)—and she naturally moves into a more serene state of equilibrium. The difficult ups and downs that can come with menstruation are left behind. No monthly bleeding to deal with is a great liberation and not something to be feared as some kind of intrinsic loss. Instead, the continuum of love and lovemaking can now go on undisturbed by the monthly onset of ovulation and menstruation. And most of all, it is very liberating to no longer have to worry about birth control.

Tantric Inspiration

And this is my observation—that if grownups are a little more meditative, children imbibe the spirit very easily. They are so sensitive. They learn whatsoever is there in the atmosphere; they learn the vibe of it. They never bother about what you say. What you are—they always respect that. And they have a very deep perceptivity, a clarity, an intuitiveness. You may be smiling but they will immediately know that it is false, because your eyes will be saying something else—and more than that your whole body will be saying something else—that you are angry, that you are just pretending, that it is just a policy.

They may not be able to formulate it in so many words, but they immediately feel it. So never be untrue with children because they will immediately know it. And once a child comes to know that his parents are untrue, his whole trust is lost. That is his first trust in life, his very base, and if that is lost he will become a skeptic. Then he cannot trust anybody. He cannot trust life, he cannot trust God, because those things are very far away things. Even the father deceived, even the mother deceived; even they were not reliable, so what to say of anything else now?

Once a child learns . . . and every child is going to learn; it is impossible to deceive a child. There is no method discovered up to now on how to deceive a child. He simply knows where you are, who you are. It is intuitive, it has nothing to do with his intellect. In fact the more intellectual he will become, the more he will lose this intuitiveness, and he will not be able to see things as they are. Right now a child is immediate. He simply looks through and through. He looks at you and you are transparent. So never be deceptive.

Love him and allow him to be a little meditative and much is possible.

OSHO, TRANSCRIBED TEACHINGS,
THE PASSION FOR THE IMPOSSIBLE

Tantric Meditation
Radiating Love

It is advantageous to take some time to practice love on your own. Sit upright in a comfortable position, alone in your room for about thirty minutes. Close your eyes and bring your awareness to your heart/breasts, and feel yourself to be loving. Radiate love from your heart and imagine that you fill the whole room with your expanding love energy. Soon you will feel yourself vibrating with a new frequency. If you feel yourself swaying, as if you are a wave in the great ocean of love, allow it. Let your whole room be filled with love. Intentionally create vibrations of love energy around you, and you may start to feel that something around your body is changing. It can feel like a warmth rising around your body, like a deep orgasm. You will feel yourself becoming more alive. If you feel moved to dance or sing to express your love, allow it. Through meditating on love you are likely to experience that you are the source of love, and not—as you have always thought—that love comes from somebody else. When you are able to connect to the love within yourself, it is a preparation for transforming your lover into a person with the right receptivity for you.

12

Tantric Orgasm and Same-Sex Partners

*T*his letter came to me in e-mail form during the final days of completing this manuscript.

I happened upon your Web site while doing some investigation on tantric sex. I think you have an excellent Web site and especially found the excerpts from the book to be interesting and informative. However, I have a question related to tantric sex and everything I have read about it so far.

First, let me give you a bit of background. I have been in a relationship with a man for over fourteen years. We stopped having sex several years ago—not by my choice, but by his. He is not interested in sex and nothing I have done to try and change the situation has helped. He refuses to see a counselor or go to any workshops, and simply accepts the "fact" that he has a low sex drive. Even when we were having sex, it was infrequent and not very satisfactory, despite my attempts to try different techniques to get him interested. He assures me that his lack of drive has nothing to do with his love for me and I know he does not seek other partners.

A few years ago, I ended up—out of desperation—having an affair with another woman. It was not something I sought out necessarily, though I was vulnerable and had at times in my life felt attractions to women. What I discovered through this affair was that, for me, sex with a woman was much more pleasurable than I had ever experienced with a man. The reason was that it was not "goal oriented" sex and had more to do with sensual pleasure. Often, my female partner and I never had orgasms, but would make love for hours. Of course, I recognize that I could just as easily have had a female partner who had bought into the idea of sex being all about the orgasm. I think this is how we are socialized in Western cultures and therefore even lesbians buy into this view.

When I began reading about tantric sex, it brought to mind my affair and my feelings about lesbian sex. It seemed to me that two women are more likely to naturally practice a more tantric style of sex, because we are more sensual (and I know we could argue that this, too, is related to the way women are socialized). However, I noticed that there is very little written about homosexual sex as it pertains to tantric practices. It seems most of the reputable tantric Web sites are extremely heterosexually oriented. My attempts to find anything on tantric sex for lesbians lead me mostly to pornographic Web sites or to workshops for lesbians with nothing written on the topic. And, although I remain in my chaste, heterosexual relationship, I identify myself as bisexual and would like to see more balance. Is there a reason that most of the books are for heterosexuals? Is it related somehow to the spiritual origins of tantric practices that perhaps don't allow for homosexual love? I am just curious—and I'm not sure you have the answers, but I am sure there are many gay and lesbian people out there wondering the same thing.

This is only one of several messages that I have received over the last few years asking me the same question: what about tantra and homosexuals? It is sometimes also asked during my heterosexual couple workshops, because most people have a homosexual sibling or friend. While I cannot say I have confirmed answers, I do have insights into how tantric principles can be applied between bodies of the same sex. My own tantric exploration has been within the heterosexual sphere, although every hug I share with a person is a tantric moment, be it a man or woman.

For many of us, exploring sexuality with a same-sex partner is part of a progression of natural sexual development. Human sexuality makes its first appearance in an auto-erotic way, in the exploration of the pleasures of one's own genitals in early childhood. This will usually change within a few years into a curiosity about the genitals of others of the same sex (homosexuality). There can also be a simultaneous interest in the genitals of the opposite sex, hence the ubiquitous "doctors and nurses" games that children create intentionally to explore each other's genitals. The actual attraction to the opposite sex (heterosexuality) for the purposes of sexual intercourse comes as a later, third, phase.

Society frowns upon and discourages innocent sexual interaction between children in their search to know themselves. Part of this is because it often happens between siblings, due to their proximity to each other, and the fear is that it will foster incestuous relationships. When we as children are discovered while attempting to fulfil our sexual curiosity, we get punished, made to feel we have done something wrong, made to feel guilty about the pleasure we have elicited from our genitals. If we manage to get away with it undiscovered, we nevertheless feel guilty for having done something secretly and therefore wrongly. Through fear of sex and lack of understanding of true sexuality, the sexual/life energy becomes repressed in each of us.

For some people, exploration with the same sex can extend into teenage years through the forced separation of the sexes, as in unisex boarding schools. Monasteries or other institutions that hold men and women apart will automatically encourage sexual exploration with the same sex. As the basic life force, sex is a drive that demands expression. What matters is whom you choose—or who is available—to consummate this expression with.

For survival we are designed to reproduce, which makes heterosexuality the next step in human sexual expression. (There *is* a fourth stage, at which an exceptional individual fully transcends sex through having embraced its elements deeply and then lives in twenty-four-hour ecstasy.)

Many people in later years, especially women, will opt totally out of sex because it fails to satisfy. (For some men this is a less easy choice, hence the many perverse ways some men release their sexual frustrations.) Women easily become autosexual again, or they become asexual, avoiding their own genitals completely. Some women deliberately choose a same-sex partner or find themselves emerging with an attraction to their same sex. A couple of lesbian women have told me that they felt they were born lesbian and were never really interested in males at any time. In fact, they were attracted to other girls before they even knew what sexual attraction was. There can be many reasons for abstention, just as there can be for the homosexual option.

But as I see the situation at present, for countless generations now we have been without positive reflection of man's and woman's sexual potential and the love that is so created. This lack of example is due to the very misunderstanding of sex itself, the theme of earlier chapters. As things stand, in the absence of guidance or insight into sexual expression, it can be easier to avoid the challenge presented by the unknown opposite sex (a complex challenge, given the level of sexual misunderstanding). Instead one can choose either to abstain from sexual contact completely, or to stay with the same sex because that sex is known and understood, since it is also a part of oneself.

Awareness of Present Moment, Relaxation, Sensitivity

If I were to simply divide the tantric approach in half, there would be a) the essential aspect of the so-called present moment, and b) the essential aspect of bodies existing as equal and opposite forces. As far as the first aspect goes, any two people, homosexual or heterosexual, can be increasingly more present to each other, more in and down in the body and aware of themselves, and thus more sensitive to their partners, their children, their parents. The more physically close we are, as in the case of lovers, the greater the opportunity to practice awareness and create the present between us. For same-sex partners, as with heterosexuals, the tantric principles apply all the way.

Tantra tells us to be aware of what we do and how we do it, to unhook slowly from excitement and drift toward relaxation, to practice being here and now and not so pinpointed on a goal. The implication is that for *all* lovers the effort is toward *not* using the genitals solely for climax purposes. The attempt is still to retain the energy so that it can spread through the body and empower the body, and to avoid the repeated discharge of life energy. It continues to mean that love should be a meditation rather than an activity.

For any two people, eye contact—using receptive soft vision as described in chapter 2—will profoundly intensify the meeting, as will relaxing into orgasm, as discussed in detail in chapter 9. Slowing down in any or all movements will enhance the experience tremendously. Consciously breathing will expand your body energies beautifully. Kissing deeply with the lips adds intimacy and intensity. Any awareness, and the challenge that comes with it, creates a bond, a sense of a unifying force encompassing greater intimacy and love. This happens because awareness transforms sex into love. And love is what we are all longing to receive and to give. Presence, silence, stillness, the essence of meditation and relaxation can be developed as a heart-opening link between any two people. Even a person alone will benefit from more inner awareness, more stillness and relaxation, meditation, less focus on the goal in any daily activities, less doing and more being in the here and now, enjoying the moment.

Opposite Polarities and Genital Correspondence

Many of the guidelines listed above can be used with equal effect by both heterosexual lovers and homosexual lovers. However, most of the guidelines for sexual intercourse pertain to heterosexuals and will therefore not apply. Nevertheless, the information can be of value in reconceiving how one goes about genital intercourse, and why. Heterosexual guidelines do not apply because of the sameness of the genitals in same-sex partners: the genitals do not correspond with each other and fit one into the other. The genitals are equal but they are not opposite; instead of a hand in a glove there is a glove and a glove, or a hand and a hand.

Tantra is based on the union of male and female aspects as equal and

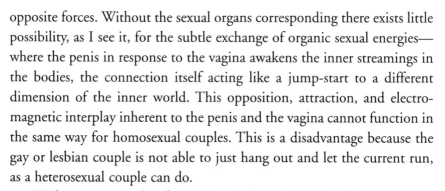

opposite forces. Without the sexual organs corresponding there exists little possibility, as I see it, for the subtle exchange of organic sexual energies—where the penis in response to the vagina awakens the inner streamings in the bodies, the connection itself acting like a jump-start to a different dimension of the inner world. This opposition, attraction, and electromagnetic interplay inherent to the penis and the vagina cannot function in the same way for homosexual couples. This is a disadvantage because the gay or lesbian couple is not able to just hang out and let the current run, as a heterosexual couple can do.

With women couples, for example, where the overall polarity is feminine, there will be a meeting of two receptive genitals, negative with negative (vagina-vagina) and positive with positive (heart/breasts-heart/breasts) instead of vice versa, positive to negative, which completes the circuit. The absence of the tantric aspect of genital correspondence in homosexual sex requires a complete re-viewing of the genitals and how to use them in applying tantric principles to create higher states. The first shift is already mentioned in the previous section: a stepping away from stimulation and excitement to discover ways of containing the sexual energy and so inviting it to rise upward, not discharging it.

The same challenges of moving away from one's sexual conditioning apply to homosexuals as to heterosexuals. Perhaps it might be more difficult, especially for gay men, to find a passive, more feminine way of being with each other's genitals, instead of constantly seeking intensity of sensation. The problem with excessive stimulation is that it makes the genitals insensitive; they begin to lose their capacity to feel, and slowly nothing turns you on any more, the old tricks don't seem to work. Then there is a need and desire for more and more stimulation, which in some cases can leave a person feeling quite numb to himself. The inner sensitivities have been blasted with an overdose of sensation. Sensitivity arises with awareness, so when we use our bodies insensitively to satisfy our sexual minds, we are closing ourselves down to our inner treasures. The guideline for any couple interested in tantra, homosexual or heterosexual, is always to seek sensitivity rather than sensation. Sensation dulls while sensitivity awakens inner sources of delight and pleasure.

The Auto-Ecstatic Individual

Having stated clearly the genital need of equal and opposite forces as essential to tantra, I remind you now that our basic inner set-up is bisexual. This is indeed the very foundation of tantra. Each one of us contains male and female poles, which makes each individual essentially auto-ecstatic. It seems rather obvious, then, that there has always been and will always be a variety of sexual expressions among human beings. In the homosexual connection, the inherent potential of the sexual situation is limited, first because reproduction is not possible, and second because of the lack of alignment in polarity. But I am certain that the ultimate potential of the individual is not affected, because ultimately the source of orgasmic states lies within each person; it is an inner celebration of the male and female elements. So it becomes more a question of how we get there, how we awaken our inner ecstatic potential. In homosexuality and heterosexuality the routes are similar and at the same time diverse.

On my way to deliver the completed manuscript of this book to the publisher, I fortunately and unexpectedly met a friend who then sent me the following report about her experiences with sex.

A woman shares her experience: "My entire life I have been bisexual. Sex used to be frustrating with both the sexes. This temporary fit of ecstasy left me almost always feeling empty afterward. So I was insatiable, a true nymphomaniac. Then many years ago I participated in a group with Diana—we called it 'The Tantra Experiment.' It changed my view and experience of sex completely. Here I was practicing how to *not* run with my hormones and lust, learning to relax into sex. Nothing really tantric was happening yet, but mysteriously it was the most fulfilling sex I had ever had. After that I was only interested in tantric lovemaking, which at that point only happened with men. When a woman crossed my path I would have a short fling, but I did not want to go back to what I called 'doing' sex.

"Everything changed when I met my female partner four years ago. To my great astonishment, the famous 'circle of energy' happened without genital penetration. A kiss or an embrace was enough to set off the silent implosion. My mind was like scrambled eggs. I could not comprehend it. It shattered a lot of beliefs and ideas I had about male and female. After all, the male and female reside in every human being; it seemed that we both have integrated these polarities and can rest in the silence of being and heart. This is a total energetic penetration! Sometimes one of us is more in the 'male,' outgoing energy and the circling goes in one direction. Sometimes it goes in two directions at the same time. At times it is full on and at times not. One thing is that we cannot 'do' it. Maybe there are ways to direct the energy that we are not aware of yet. In my experience, the difference between tantra with the opposite sex and tantra with a same-sex partner is that with the opposite sex the genital penetration almost always allows for the circle of energy to happen, or at least more easily. At the same time, right now I am menopausal and there is not always enough sexual energy available to allow for the tantric orgasm. The ecstatic melting then happens purely in the heart."

The Focus of Sexual Exchange for Women

As far as women go, a tantric approach means shifting away from an over-focused clitoral approach that encourages excitement and toward a style in which the breasts are loved and understood as the focal point of the female energy system. As explained in chapter 5, breasts are the source of the energy in a woman's deepest orgasm; an orgasmic state can be experienced just through deeply loving the breasts. (A woman can lavish love on her own breasts as well, to arouse herself into an expanded state.) The energy of the breasts accumulates and spreads downward, resonating in the vagina. For this there is no necessity of penetration by a penis.

Instead of going for excitement and orgasm, a lover should treat the clitoris more gently and passively, so as to create a flow of energy backward into the vagina. In fact, she should treat the vagina itself gently. Any phallic substitutes will naturally lack the electromagnetic intelligence possessed by the penis in relation to the vagina. In particular, there is perhaps less perception and sensitivity in the upper vaginal region, which is significant in deep penetration by the penis for the accessing of ecstatic energies in women. A lifeless, phallic-shaped object cannot meaningfully communicate with the receptive feminine pole; however, mechanical vibrations emanating from them can do something to awaken the more subtle energies. Fingers certainly have much more sensitivity than a vibrator but only when offered with a delicate, loving, conscious touch. There are beneficial therapeutic massage techniques that can help to release tensions that are held in the vagina and obscure its polarity. (These require personal instruction and are therefore beyond the scope of this book.) However, fingers will naturally lack the perception, finesse, and catalytic effect of the "magnetic" penis head (chapter 6). If simulating vaginal penetration, the guideline would be to do so in a fashion that steers away from friction and excessive building of excitement (resulting in more tensions). Move toward relaxation and the sustained presence of the finger(s) (short nails!) as the receptive partner absorbs, while primarily focusing on the heart and breasts. The receptive partner may feel a circling downward to the vagina that returns upward to the heart via the inner "magnetic rod." Or she can positively direct the imagination toward the inner circle of energy: breasts-vagina-breasts. In this way it is possible for a woman to experience an ecstatic state without necessarily involving a clitoral orgasm and an undue discharge of energy, just as in the case of a heterosexual woman, who may have the additional help of the penis in the vagina to open the inner channels.

Homosexual Love and the Feminist Movement

For many feminists today, the clitoris has become a symbol of woman's sexual freedom because through it woman is able to reclaim her long lost orgasm. This movement is certainly well motivated but perhaps a little misled in that what has emerged is an intensified focus on the clitoris, with a corresponding abandonment of the vagina and the receptive pole of feminine energy. The clitoris, through a buildup of excitement, is used as a "positive pole" for discharge, not as a link back into the vagina to connect with the receptive energies. With the focus on the clitoris also comes talk of multiple orgasms (which are indeed possible, and will always be a temptation); however, these are based primarily on excitement, with its consequences of tension and emotionality.

Because at present we see this major identification with the clitoris as the center of female sexuality, some feminists may view the relative de-emphasizing of the clitoris in the tantric picture as a step backward for the feminist movement, and for women in general. It is also quite possible that women who are unfamiliar with (or inexperienced in) the intrinsic power of yielding or giving way through a more absorbent and receptive approach will strongly react to my tantric suggestions on the feminist level. They may feel a resistance to giving up the male approach, which they have used in freeing themselves sexually. However, with understanding of the connection between peak orgasm and distressing states of emotionality (see chapter 10), women may see that they need to explore themselves on a different level when together as lovers.

In tantric exploration, women should avoid the temptation to go for the so-called male approach because basically it is an imitation of man, who is at this time completely unconscious in his sexual expression and by no means a reflection of the qualities of true masculine force. Trying to be like a man only makes a woman hard and tough and inaccessible. To begin with, a woman should go for being feminine and as a consequence, her *real* inner man will awaken. Naturally within any two people (heterosexual or homosexual) a certain kind of polarity can develop—one may shift to become the more responsible, worldly, doing type (positive) while the other becomes the more encompassing, loving, being type (negative)—but in sexual love with one another, women should not really attempt to copy men. Rather, two women can find the feminine way to make love by reconfiguring the essential elements.

Recently I spoke with a good friend who has many gay and lesbian couples as close friends. She told me that this is what she observes: the gay couples tend toward being more womanlike while the lesbian couples tend to being more manlike. *Both* of the partners in each couple tend toward the equal and opposite that is lacking in their couple. This can be understood as a balancing of polarities, which for sure it is in a certain sense; but unfortunately, I repeat, for a woman to be like a man is not to her ultimate advantage.

Where homosexuals are at an automatic disadvantage is in not being able to "hang out" with genitals united and let sex happen by itself, the way

that heterosexual couples can. The tantric union of male and female elements produces the current of sexual (life) energy, providing an ongoing
focus for awareness and a source of great pleasure. It is possible to sustain
hours of penetration without doing much at all. The correspondence of the
genitals encourages a "being" approach—in fact, sex presents the perfect circumstances for meditation.

In contrast, the homosexual lack of correspondence leads to a more
"doing" approach, which easily turns to excitement and peak orgasm.
Nevertheless the thrust should always be toward "being" even while a certain amount of "doing" may be required, and of course all kinds of doing
can be radically modified by using awareness, as suggested earlier in the
chapter. It is likely that female homosexuals, when they drop the orgasm-
oriented style of sex, tend toward a meditative type of sexual expression
more easily than male homosexuals, simply by virtue of their overall negative polarity.

I sent this chapter to a friend of mine who has had sexual experiences
with both men and women, asking for her comments. I am most grateful
to her for her response, which follows.

A woman shares her experience: "So, I read your chapter and I'll tell you
a little of what my experience has been. Having known the tantric way
with men, it has always been a conflict for me to be with women, knowing that the advantages of opposite polarity are not possible. However, for
many other reasons, I keep finding myself drawn to relationships with
women over and over again.

"I'm still in the search of what can or can't be done with a woman, and
I'm trying to understand a little bit more what happens energetically when
I am with a woman. I think it would take a lot more experience than what I
have to give really conclusive answers, but I have had some experiences
(one was very strong) that might give a little direction as to where to begin.

"Whether I was with a man or a woman, I had never liked being penetrated by anything other than a penis (fingers, vibrators, etc). When I had
sex with a woman, I was limited to caressing, touching, and oral sex, which
always led to orgasm because the clitoris was always involved.

"Then, with a female partner, I decided to try penetration with a finger with the specific intention of not seeking excitement and orgasm. I asked her to gently penetrate me and not move inside—a simulation of silent penetration with a penis. I could feel the two pulses, my vagina's and her finger's. It was delicious to just feel the pulsation there with no movement or stimulation. After a little while the pulses started synchronizing and it was a pretty delicious experience, with no need of excitement or orgasm at all. We did it several times and I started noticing a mini, mini, mini similarity to sensations I've had with men, very subtle energy flowing throughout the body.

"Then came the issue of still having memories in my body of having been raped as a child. As I had mentioned to you when you were in the process of writing about sexual abuse and its effects, the problem for most women in this situation is that while the polarity created by a gentle penetration by the penis is a great way to cleanse those memories from the vagina, most woman in severe trauma will not get to that point. Often they fear intimacy or they can't attract men or they have turned to relationships with women or, as a means of repeating the pattern, they end up attracting the wrong men who certainly can't be very meditative about sex. For myself, once the memory was there it was simply impossible, for several of the above reasons, to get myself into such a healing situation with a man.

"Back to the silent penetration exercise with my female partner: Once again I asked her to penetrate me gently with a finger and to not move. When the pulses started synchronizing, I asked her to start applying a very soft pressure in different directions, first up, staying there for a while with both of us in silence. And sure enough, a lot of energy started moving. Then she applied pressure on the diagonal, then to the right, and so forth—slight pressure with the whole finger. Most of the time I experienced a very silent cleansing, just feeling and breathing, while a couple of times there was a little more, crying and strong emotions coming to the surface. It was pretty unbelievable to be dealing with my past trauma it in this way.

"After we did this several times, the energy in my vagina was clearly more open and the penetration without movement became more and more pleasant. Once, I *did* have an experience that could be compared to a tantric one with a man. How that happened without the opposing polarity of the penis and vagina, god knows. It just did. It was certainly not as intense or as obvious as my experiences with men, but then again, I haven't delved into this that much.

"Clearly the first aspect of tantra, as you mention in the chapter, is the first opening for gay couples. About the second aspect and the polarity issue, the above is the only thing I can share for the moment. Maybe this approach could open a door for lesbian women. I really can't say for sure."

I have heard it suggested that in homosexual couples, the polarity of one partner can energetically shift into its opposite, so that same-sex couples will begin to internally balance each other on a polarity level. This implies that in one lesbian partner the negative vagina would shift to a positive phenomenon, and the breasts to a passive one. I am inclined to doubt this, especially in view of the fact that when a woman has a breast or her cervix removed, the magnetic phenomenon present in the physical tissues continues to exist on an energetic level.

In saying this I am aware that there is very little research done on homosexual experience, and research could perhaps prove me quite wrong. A friend recently told me that a lesbian she knows, who has been interested only in women from the beginning of her sexual life, feels that she has an "etheric penis." Perhaps something of this nature is possible without an actual change occurring in the body energy. Certainly, if she is talking about an "inner penis," which is the experience of a constantly alive magnetic rod, then I can relate to this feeling. With the current emphasis in sex being toward excitement, not toward meditation, we will need a major shift in consciousness for a reliable body of material on homosexual tantric experience to emerge in order to give substance to its practice.

Because this is a book for women, I am not saying much about gay men; however, the many principles of tantra will of course apply to them, in the sense that the energy is encouraged to stream inward and upward toward the heart (positive to negative) instead of being discharged from the positive. And not unlike the dildo/penis replacement, I do feel it is unlikely that the highly erotic zone of the anus can successfully replace the electromagnetic cavity of the vagina. (This applies also to the case of heterosexuals who take part in anal sex, although the female internal connection via the anus may perhaps be different from that of the male). It is likely that the anal approach is seldom slow and easy—that is, tantric style—but instead reflects the conventional style of going for stimulation, excitement, and ejaculation. Until the anus is not used for stimulation and eroticism, we will not know whether there is some internal, magical, electromagnetic connection to be made there.

Tantric Spiritual Background Is Heterosexual

From its origin tantra has been oriented toward heterosexuality. The subject of our study here, the so-called left hand path of tantra, uses the sexual current on a physical level for an outer union (man and woman), which leads to an inner union, which results in states of meditative ecstasy.*

In India we find a multitude of temples that are now thousands of years old (the most famous ones being in Khajuraho) containing statues of man and woman in sexual union. Usually these stone partners are maintaining some acrobatic position in which, when viewed conventionally, one cannot imagine how they achieve any kind of sex at all. But with the advantage of tantric eyes, knowing that the penetration of the vagina can be sustained for hours and produce endless delight, one sees that these statues do represent reality, positions and all! The remarkable thing about many of these statues is that you can actually see the ecstasy alive in their faces and you feel it radiating as you look at them. The people who built those temples in ancient times, especially the sculptors of the statues, were not artisans but artists, living the very experience they were creating in stone. Their personal inner experience was embodied in stone; their ecstasy is still palpable thousands of years later.

---

*The right hand path is the school of the Buddhist tantric meditation practices in which sexual energy is employed on a symbolic level; the practitioner uses visualization to stimulate the inner union.

The emphasis on heterosexuality in these spiritual practices is not due to a sexual prejudice but exists because tantric experiences arise with ease between the opposite forces of male and female. Tantric sex is the most direct and natural route to awaken the inner opposite force within oneself, the outer opposite being used to reach the inner opposite. Woman can use man to awaken her inner man. Without the genital correspondence, which in and of itself creates intense ecstatic moments, a sustained, meditative state of union for hours at a time becomes more difficult. But for sure it is not out of the question. To really explore the tantric frame as a homosexual requires deconditioning the stimulation-as-sexuality attitude and rediscovering sensitivity as a door to bliss—the same tasks required of heterosexuals.

Masturbation and Self-Love

On the question of masturbation, or self-love, once again the tantric principle applies: anything done with awareness cannot be wrong or unnatural. It is not what you do but how you do it. As always, experiment with loving yourself in a way that does not depend exclusively on excitement but on expansion of energy through relaxation. Retain the energy in your body without automatically discharging it. While masturbating, avoid unnecessary contractions in the body or in the vagina, and don't be too demanding of the clitoris. If you have an orgasm, don't force it—relax into it, take it all very slowly. The masturbation that includes more and more intense stimulation to the clitoris or vagina can slowly deaden the very sensitivity that is sought, in the end leaving not much pleasure at all.

Include the breasts in your experience. Make them the focus, make the shift away from the clitoris as you discover the new doorway to sexual expression. Stroke, caress, and expand the energy through your own body or your partner's. A woman alone, or on her own, can enhance her femininity by meditating on the breasts as suggested at the end of chapter 5. Lesbian women can use this practice to support the awakening of the orgasmic energy in the body, doing it as a separate practice or as part of foreplay. Then, during lovemaking, massage your own breasts and also show your partner how to touch your breasts. Even though with two women together there will be more knowing about how breasts feel while being touched, it is a beneficial practice to be guided by the one you love. In the same way, explore the clitoris and the surrounding area, sharing and discovering what kind of touch supports the sensations and sensitivity in your body and what distracts from your more subtle inner feelings and delicate sensations.

Applying Tantric Principles to Same-Sex Relationships

Quite a few years ago in Mexico City I had the opportunity to work with a group of nine gay couples who were all HIV positive. I was given the concluding day with them as the grand finale of a six-month-long intensive healing program that included meditation and natural therapies, which had assisted their physical and psychological conditions tremendously. I was invited for the final wrap-up because the therapist wished for the men to be left with a positive impression about sex. Most of them had really disastrous sexual backgrounds and exceptionally negative imprints about sex, as well as a sexually transmitted disease to top it off. In these painful and challenging circumstances it was not easy for them to view sex with any feelings of contentment or joy.

As at that point I had never imagined applying tantra to homosexual couples, I at first balked at the invitation from my friend, the therapist. After some thought, I told her that I would present the aspect of tantra that pertains to inner awareness and creating the present moment. I would not, however, be willing to explain the picture of the innate polarities and how the male-female interaction is conceived by nature. But my friend was insistent—I was to give the complete picture—and I reluctantly agreed, not really seeing the point of it.

The morning was a beautiful experience. Leading the male couples through a structure that brought them into the present moment with each other, I saw before my eyes a profound transformation that turned out to be a great teaching for me: a conscious, sensitive merging into each other; relaxing into the now of the body; melting into tender, powerful hugs. Silence and sincerity and love filled the air. It was so touching that at times I had tears in my eyes, as did many of the men themselves.

At the end of the morning one man shared the wish that he had found this space, or known how to find it, with his lover years earlier. It would have made all the difference; and now it was late for it, given the knowledge that he was nearing the end of his life.

After a break for lunch, we resumed in the afternoon with a discussion of the male-female polarities, the interaction of the penis and vagina, the breasts, and erection. The information was received with much interest and I felt and saw no resistance at all among the men. We finished with a meditation imagining the energy circles in our own bodies, then had tearful, loving farewells before going our separate ways.

This impressive experience gave me the authority to say that *all* couples, regardless of gender, definitely have positive, inspiring experiences when they use tantric principles during intimacy. Every couple can benefit from being more aware and relaxed when making love, and all human bodies have both positive and negative polarities within them. As more homosexual couples experiment with tantra, I look forward to their feedback on how they have put these ideas into practice to engender successful and loving relationships.

Tantric Inspiration

Man has to transcend sex, whatsoever kind of sex it is, because unless you go beyond your biology you will never know your soul. Meanwhile—before you go beyond—it is your freedom to be whatsoever you want to be.

Don't make a problem out of it. Nothing has to be done about it. I don't tackle individual problems. My whole approach is that there are millions of diseases and only one cure and that cure is meditation.

You meditate—homosexual, heterosexual, bisexual . . . You meditate. Become more still and more silent. Create inner emptiness. Become more transparent. And then things will start changing. You will be able to see what you are doing to yourself. And if it is right you will go on doing it with more joy, with more totality, with more intensity, with more passion. And if it is wrong it will simply drop, just like dead leaves falling from a tree. So I cannot suggest any specific method because to me all the problems are arising because we have become minds and we have forgotten that deep down there is a space within us which can be called no-mind. Entering that space, no-mind, will give you perspective, vision, clarity.

Meditate. Sit silently watching your thoughts—homosexual, heterosexual, whatsoever they are, it doesn't matter. You watch, you become the witness. Slowly, slowly a distance will be created between you and your thoughts. And one day suddenly—the realization that you are not your mind. And that day a revolution has happened within you. After that day you will never be the same again. A transcendence will have happened.

OSHO, TRANSCRIBED TEACHINGS,
THE BOOK OF THE BOOKS, VOLUME 9

Tantric Meditation
The Golden Flower

Do this meditation early in the morning or when you are going to sleep at night.

Lie down comfortably in your bed, on your back, with about half an hour to yourself. Relax for a few minutes with your eyes closed. When you breathe in, begin to visualize great light entering from your head into your body, as if a sun has just risen close to your head—golden light pouring into your head, as if you are hollow and golden light is pouring in at the top and going deeper and deeper, all the way down and out through your toes. As you breathe out, visualize darkness entering through your toes, a great dark river entering through your toes, traveling all the way up and out through your head.

Do slow, deep breathing so you can visualize this. Go very slowly. Breathing in, let golden light come into you through the top of your head; it is here that the Golden Flower opens. The golden light will cleanse your whole body and will fill it with creativity. This is male energy. When you exhale, you let darkness, the deepest darkness you can conceive, like a dark night, come from your toes upward like a river, and out through your head. This is feminine energy. It soothes you and makes you receptive. It calms you and gives you rest. Then inhale again and let the golden light enter in. Keep breathing in this manner for about twenty minutes and then relax after that for another ten minutes.

You can do this early in the morning, when you just start to wake and are still wavering between sleep and waking. Right there, start the process of breathing in the light and breathing out darkness for twenty minutes. If you do the meditation at night and you fall asleep doing it, the impact will remain in the subconscious and will go on working. After a three-month period you will begin to notice that the energy that was constantly building up and concentrating itself in the sex center is no longer gathering there. The energy is going upward; the energy begins rising by itself.

Conclusion
Embracing Our True Feminine Power

With the unmasking of woman's true role in sex and the profound implications of true femininity, it is possible that you will find contradictory feelings arising simultaneously—an uplifting sense of inspiration or empowerment along with the heaviness of feeling overwhelmed and intimidated by new input, daunted and unsure about how to proceed, how to alter the way of making love *in reality*. Rather than getting bogged down in all the pros and cons, simply take immediate action by starting to refocus on the body right away. Even this very second, while sitting and reading, relax the jaw and shoulders, the belly. Enjoy two or three nice deep breaths as the pleasure of a physical letting go spreads through you. Or rest with your awareness in the breasts and nipples for the next few minutes, sensing them from within, radiating warmth outward. Close the eyes and enjoy feeling rooted in your body; it is the link to your being, a natural bridge to the endless source of love residing within you.

Shifting awareness from mind to body, as you have just done and as you are encouraged to do by the tantric meditations offered at the end of each chapter, will gradually have an impact on your body. As sensitivity increases, subtle yet powerful shifts will be detectable in your energy system. Shifts of awareness back and down into the body can be done at will at any time. In place of being caught up in the endless circling train of thoughts, begin directing attention inward, merging internally with any pleasant sensations present in your body. The next time you embrace your lover or make love, make similar shifts of awareness, from the outer to the inner. Start out innocently; be childlike, stepping to the side of the known sexual you, and sink into your body. This instantly creates a more relaxed unhurried "tantric" state of being, without the pressure of big goals and expectations clouding the simple reality of two human bodies together. Take small experimental steps each time you make love or hug (porously) or kiss (lingeringly). While hugging, caressing, kissing become merged with the experience of *how* you are doing it, so that the whole experience evolves in graceful slow motion, choreographed by inner awareness. Experiment with some of the guidelines given in the earlier chapters, then attempt others, then begin putting together various combinations according to what your experience reveals to you.

You will find it advantageous to play with reducing excitement, thereby reducing the urges for conventional orgasm, and losing the creative potential of lovemaking. Introducing awareness allows you to move into the encounter in a sensual catlike way, connected to what is happening as it is happening. Let it be a mobilization of all your senses. Intensify your awareness of your vagina; consciously transform its quality into a receptive channel, instilling it with an absorbent, drinking quality, which is enticing, alluring, inviting, available, and welcoming to the male force. Also bring the breasts into awareness and see what impact this has on your responses. What deepens your yes; what reduces your yes? What expands your body energy; what causes a shrinking? What heightens sensitivity; what deadens sensitivity? Pursue any avenues that interest to you in particular. For instance, if the clitoris is a place you emphasize, experiment with including it in a more relaxed undemanding way or leaving it out or leaving it to later. The inner attitude should be investigative, rather than being an attitude of impatient expectation or demand for immediate results. Instead, cultivate an attitude of observation, standing back and challenging routine patterns, then witness what happens. As an outcome, you will gradually establish the truth in yourself. It is a challenge to confront oneself in this way, let me not lull you into thinking it necessarily effortless. Of course it takes an effort to break away from the past but it is the effort of being aware, not the effort of doing. In time it becomes less and less effort to remain rooted in the body; one is simply present with joy.

In the process of bringing awareness to habitual, unconscious sexual habits a gradual inner transformation takes place. You will emerge with new eyes, new values, new insights, indeed you will view and experience all of life from another perspective. Reinventing yourself as a woman or arriving at your femininity anew will be the result of a slow, steady pursuit. By following an inner inquiry you embrace the willingness to reveal a deeper layer of yourself to yourself. Osho encourages us in this way:

And this merger [sex] should not become unconscious, otherwise you miss the point. Then it is a beautiful sex act, but not transformation. It is beautiful, nothing is wrong in it, but it is not transformation. And if it is unconscious then you will always be moving in a rut. Again and again you will want to have this experience. The experience is beautiful as far as it goes, but it will become a routine. And each time you have it, again more desire is created. The more you have it, the more you desire it, and you move in a vicious circle. You don't grow, you just rotate.

Rotation is bad, because then growth is not happening. Then energy is simply wasted. Even if the experience is good, the energy is wasted, because much more was possible. And it was just at the corner, just a turn, and much more was possible. With the same energy the divine could have been achieved. With the same energy the ultimate ecstasy is possible, and you are wasting that energy in momentary experiences. And by and by those experiences will become boring, because repeated again and again, everything becomes a boring thing. When the newness is lost, boredom is created.

If you remain alert you will see: first, changes of energy in the body; second, dropping of the thoughts from the mind; and third, dropping of the ego from the heart. And when this third thing has happened, your energy, that sex energy has become meditative energy.[1]

Doubts can easily surface and dampen our creative and courageous responses to the truth. Mind, with its many voices, will begin with excuses to put us off taking action now, encouraging us into postponement. Doubts are triggered by our fear of the unknown, a fear of standing naked, stripped of our stylized skills and strategies, and a deep fear that our control will be lost. However, witnessing instills a new control, the control of the witnessing self, the control that arises through awareness. This type of control is so natural that you never ever feel that you are controlling. In reality, through understanding and experiencing the feminine body from a new perspective, woman will not be devalued or depreciated in any way. In fact this new awareness is a tremendous empowerment.

When we (man and woman) learn to understand one another's psychology and physiology, we can embrace our biology and our spirituality as one. With a multidimensional quality to it, sex has a far deeper significance than the production of children. It is also fun; it is play; it is prayer; it is meditation; it is a merging into oneness, into love; it is true spirituality.

For many a man (as he knows himself now), sex is not a spiritual phenomenon but only a physiological release, more in the direction of an emotional release of pent up tensions and feelings. For women sex is always, to large extent, a spiritual phenomenon, which is why women easily feel offended in sex. Unless love happens as part of a greater spiritual experience she has trouble opening up to it. Participation in loveless sex is the precise reason that so many millions of women have completely forgotten what orgasm means. Women have become sexually repressed due to man's nonunderstanding of the difference between the sexes. But it is not man's fault, personally; he too is a by-product of the social, sexual misunderstanding in force today.

The tragedy of this repression of woman and her sexual power is that whenever man's and woman's real nature is not allowed to go according to its inner needs it turns sour, becomes poisoned, crippled, or paralyzed; it can even become perverted. If woman is corrupted by man, man himself cannot remain natural either. After all, the woman gives birth to the man. If woman, as mother, does not express her sexuality naturally, her children will not learn a natural expression either. Woman certainly needs a great liberation but not through imitation of man, not through being equal to man by being exactly like him. Instead, woman's true liberation will come through being an authentic and opposite force to man.

It is an undeniably painful reality that today millions of women on Earth continue to be dominated by male sexual unconsciousness, subjected to all kinds of inhumanity, humiliation, and aggression, suffering untold emotional and physical pain as part of daily living. For these unfortunate women the fine tuning of "feminine energy," is the remotest of their concerns because, tragically, reality is dominated by the sheer struggle for survival. As women from a more privileged sector of society (which we are if holding this book in our hands) we can join our hearts in the silence of prayer, willing days of peace, love and balance to manifest on Earth. Any change in the global sexual situation cannot be dependant on a mass solution. It needs to emerge from individual consciousnesses and spread outward into the collective consciousness in true homeopathic fashion. Each woman, through understanding herself more intimately, has the capacity and power to transform her living situation into one that is satisfying and nourishing to her, thereby passing higher values down the generational line.

Returning full circle to the introduction of the book, we, as women from the privileged sector of society, are in a position to be responsible to ourselves for creating love and not letting things run on lovelessly as they have for hundreds of years. Never underestimate our intrinsic power as female members of the species. Women are very powerful people, not in the muscular sense but as far as their resistance is concerned, their life energy is concerned, their sex energy is concerned, their tolerance is concerned. Woman's whole functioning is intrinsically graceful, insightful, loving, compassionate. Henceforth woman should not rely on permission or cooperation from man before taking experimental steps to find her true self through sex. Try things out, in and out of bed, independent of your partner and what he thinks or expects or wants. Observe what happens within yourself and between yourself and your partner on an energy level. If your man is worth his salt his response will follow your lead, trusting and sensing the capacity for natural authority that all women have in sex when given the chance.

Since time immemorial women have been a collective force in healing, wisdom, and spiritual evolution but in this technological age we have become emotionally confused and have lost contact with our feminine truth. Feminine growth requires the willingness to feel anything and everything, including old and painful emotions, which often have less to do with the present than with the past. Recalling the difference between a feeling and an emotion is one of the most helpful keys in living a joyful, loving life. Remember, emotions themselves are not wrong but where we put the blame can be wrong, and damaging. Conquering states of emotionality, getting to the root of the emotions by expressing the feelings hiding behind them, and handling emotions in a conscious way is a powerful gift to creating inner balance. It is a step in maturity. Succumbing continually to upsurges of emotion keeps us in a childish frame to which the unfulfilled past keeps coming back in cycles, spilling over into the now in seismic upheavals.

Woman can begin to cut away from the myth that she is basically emotional, unstable, and given to bouts of moodiness. At the personality level, we as women have "learned" to be emotional, but emotion is not an aspect of woman's essential nature. The heart—at the center of our true being—knows only one language and that is the language of love. When searching and longing for love, it is very easy to lose oneself in the other, thereby unconsciously and accidentally giving up the power and grace of our feminine birthright. By opening consciously to man, inviting him in, while at the same time remaining true to our own feminine awareness, we transform sex between man and woman into love—a sublimely spiritual experience.

I leave you with these final words from Osho:

> Remember this: Tantra is a love effort towards existence. That is why so much of sex has been used by Tantra: because it is a love technique. It is not only love between man and woman; it is love between you and existence, and for the first time existence becomes meaningful to you through a woman. If you are a woman, then existence becomes for the first time meaningful to you through a man.[2]

Appendix
The Sympto-Thermal Method of Fertility Awareness

*W*hen a woman wishes to become intimate with her own fertility cycle, for contraception or for conception, possibly her best bet is to learn the Sympto-Thermal Method.* The brief introduction contained here should familiarize you with the method, but please do not consider it as definitive. It explains the basics of how the method works, but space doesn't permit a thorough explanation of all the possible exceptions to the rule that should be considered if you want to use the method for truly reliable birth control. If you would like to give the Sympto-Thermal method a serious try, please consult the Web site mentioned below for further guidance.

Instructions in this method are available worldwide. The SymptoTherm Foundation in Switzerland offers addresses and contact information for

---

*Contributors to the Sympto-Thermal Method information contained herein are R. Harri Wettstein, Ph.D., M.B.A., M.A., Director of Bioself SA, Geneva, Switzerland and secretary of the SymptoTherm Foundation, Morges, Switzerland; and Christine Bourgeois, president of the SymptoTherm Foundation.

the main organizations that teach this method on its Web site: www.symptotherm.ch. Each organization has its own competent network of counselors. For beginners, the SymptoTherm Foundation recommends the Bioself fertility indicator (www.bioself.com) as an educational tool, together with a good textbook about the method.

The Sympto-Thermal Method was developed by Catholic researchers in the early 1950s. The term was coined by Professor Josef Rötzer, an Austrian doctor who was one of its pioneers. Many universities are still conducting clinical and scientific research on this method, but its present form of practice has about twenty years of solid experience and statistical data testifying to its safety.

The original motive for the development of this practice was to find a "natural" alternative to so-called artificial contraception (which is prohibited by the Vatican) in order to enable Catholic couples to enjoy sex during infertile days, at times when pregnancy was not advised or desired. Paradoxically, the Fertility Awareness Method (FAM) schools and other secular organizations are indebted to the Catholic Natural Family Planning Institute, with which they do not agree on the issue of condom use. Thus, strict Natural Family Planning use of the method always implies periods of abstinence, whereas FAM has nothing against protected sex during the fertile phase. But FAM also recognizes that the use of a contraceptive device (condom, cervical cap, diaphragm) during fertile parts of the cycle diminishes contraceptive safety, and suggests that a contraceptive be used in conjunction with the Sympto-Thermal Method to prevent any failure.

The word *sympto-thermal,* as it relates to ovulation, means that there is (a) a temperature rise, indicating the passing of an egg (ovulation). This rise is always interpreted in relation to (b) observation of the cervical fluid, which also reveals ovarian activity. Other observations, such as breast tenderness and intermenstrual pain (e.g., a few sharp shooting pains associated with ovulation), can also help a woman attune to her cycle and become aware of when she is fertile and when she is not. The Sympto-Thermal Method always uses two signs—body temperature and vaginal secretions—and then "cross checks" them against each other.

How the Sympto-Thermal Cross-Check Works

A woman's monthly cycle, starting with the first day of her menstrual period as day one, will continue with some six infertile days and then enter into the fertile phase until after ovulation. Ovulation will occur near the middle of the cycle, but there is considerable variation in the exact timing of ovulation from one woman to another. With careful observation, over time a woman can become familiar with the pattern of her cycle and know when to expect ovulation each month. To be safe, she must consider herself fertile for several days preceding and following ovulation. However, by observing her waking body temperature and her cervical mucus, a woman can confirm ovulation and know when she has entered the second, absolutely infertile phase of her cycle.

Determining the Peak Day

To determine the beginning of the postovulation infertile phase, a woman first must learn to spot the *peak day*: this is *the day of her most fertile cervical fluid.* The most fertile fluid, or mucus, looks and feels like clear, slippery, uncooked egg whites. It is very elastic and can be stretched into a long string between finger and thumb without breaking—in contrast to the sticky, opaque infertile mucus that breaks immediately when thumb and forefinger are pulled apart. Once a woman has observed fertile mucus, she can pinpoint her peak day of fertility by noting the first day that the mucus quality changes drastically and begins to dry out—that is, the peak day can only be identified for sure by mucus changes the day after. That last day of slippery mucus should be considered the peak day.

A woman must observe the quality of her cervical fluid until she can identify it precisely. It might take her several cycles to really become familiar with her own peak symptoms. Each month she will record her peak day in her personal calendar or note it in the special chart provided in the manual. Her peak day may be the ovulation day. This is especially probable if she has on that day what some 10 percent of all women can feel—a few spasms of penetrating ache in the belly. This ache occurs on the side of the abdomen where the ovulating ovary lies.

According to scientific studies done by ultrasound tests with women who do not feel this kind of ache, there remains a 10 to 20 percent chance that ovulation occurs up to three days before or three days after the peak day. The minimal fertility window must take account of these six days of possible fertility. Because the egg lives for approximately eighteen hours after ovulation, and because sperm cells can survive for up to five or six days in the cervical crypts and folds, the fertility window generally extends to a minimum of eight days. Irregular cycles require extra vigilance.

Once the woman has spotted her peak day and noted it in her personal calendar or her cycle chart, she counts *until the evening of the third day* to fix the most probable end of her fertility. For example, let's say Wednesday is the peak day. She counts Thursday as the first day (it is also the day of her peak-day verification) and Friday as the second. She may expect infertility to begin the evening of the third day—Saturday evening in this example. How can she be absolutely sure about this forecast? By using the second sign, the temperature, as verification on Saturday morning.

Confirming Ovulation with Temperature

When practicing the sympto-thermal method a woman learns to observe her waking body temperature as a cross-check to her cervical mucus observations of fertility. To get an accurate reading of her waking temperature, she should take her temperature right after she wakes up in the morning. (It's okay go to the bathroom before taking the temperature or even to make tantric love *while* taking it, but excessive activity should be avoided before getting a reading.) For the first (estrogen-dominated) part of her cycle, a woman's waking body temperature will be slightly lower than her temperature after ovulation. Once ovulation has occurred, the waking temperature will rise slightly, due to a higher proportion of the hormone progesterone in the woman's body. So a woman can confirm the occurrence of ovulation by noticing when her waking temperature goes up. When a woman has observed three elevated waking temperatures—at least 0.2°C higher—following at least *six* of the lower temperatures, she will know that she has entered the infertile phase of her cycle and that she will remain infertile until her next menstruation, when her new cycle begins.

Only an adequate temperature rise can certify that the ovulation process is completely finished and that the absolutely infertile (progesterone) phase of the cycle has been established. (Such minute changes in temperature can be read only by special thermometers known as basal body temperature thermometers. The Bioself indicator [see page 208 for contact information for the Director of the Bioself company] is a most convenient and reliable tool for measuring temperature changes relative to the ovulation cycle.)

Exceptions

Occasionally the third high temperature may occur one or two days before the peak-day forecast would suggest (Thursday or Friday rather than Saturday, in our example here); in other words, the temperature rises before the peak day. (The Bioself indicator shows green too early.) It is then the viscosity of the cervical fluid that indicates Saturday evening as the beginning of the infertile phase. This cross-check determines the end of fertility fixed by the peak plus three days. This exception is very rare.

The following exception is more common. It is not risky, but it does extend the the fertile phase.

Let's continue with the same example. This time, the temperature does not rise immediately after the peak day, so that, on Saturday morning, the third high temperature is still not there. (The Bioself indicator shows red.) On Sunday morning, however, the fourth day after peak, the third high temperature is confirmed (the Bioself indicator shows green); thus, the absolute infertile days start Sunday evening, the fourth day after peak day.

The principle of cross-checking at work in these two exceptions, as everywhere, is this: *You always have to respect the fertility sign that comes last.*

What if the Bioself indicator still does not show green on Sunday or Monday morning? This means that ovulation *did not occur* and that the woman can expect another ovulation development with a *second peak day.* A woman can have two or more peak days especially when under stress. It is always the *last* peak that begins the count to the second, postovulatory phase. However, if the last peak day is not followed by the temperature rise before the next bleeding, the woman has had an anovulatory cycle.

In such situations, the woman fortunately can apply a general rule:

From the fourth evening after the peak day, whatever happens to the temperature curve (the Bioself indicator will continuously show red), the woman can consider herself as *relatively* infertile, as she is in the beginning of her cycle. The couple can safely have unprotected sex in the evening of every dry day while the woman daily keeps an eye on any potential new ovulation activity, indicated by the start of cervical fluid secretion. If the cycle remains anovulatory until the next bleeding, the woman might have an ovulation hidden by this bleeding. Only the temperature rise can confirm or refute this supposition.

Is Cross-Checking Always Needed?

Cross checking is only needed to screen out the exceptions noted earlier in this section. Once the woman really masters all fertility signs, according to her experience and her needs (provided her cycles remain strictly within the same pattern), she may concentrate on a single-sign approach: only the cervical fluid observation or only the temperature observation. But in doing this she may diminish the contraceptive safety provided by the cross-checking.

This, in a nutshell, is all a woman needs to know if she wants her sexuality to make friends with her fertility. The Sympto-Thermal Method also works during breast-feeding and perimenopause; it has its place in all types of cycles, during all gynecological ages. Using the Bioself indicator is the easiest way to learn and to manage this method.

Notes

Owing to the existence of a number of earlier editions of Osho's books, the author has provided the relevant chapter number instead of the page number for Osho references. The most recent publication details have been used.

Author's Introductory Note

1. Osho, *The Tantra Experience* (Pune, India: Rebel Publishing House, 1998) and Rufus C. Camphausen, *The Yoni: Sacred Symbol of Female Creative Power* (Rochester. Vt.: Inner Traditions, 1996).

Chapter 2

1. See Osho's *Fly without Wings, Walk without Feet and Think without Mind* (Full Circle Publishing, Ltd., 2000), chapter 5, question 3.
2. Mantak Chia, *Awaken Healing Energy through the Tao* (Santa Fe, N.M.: Aurora Press, 1983).

Chapter 4

1. Osho, *The Book of Secrets,* (New York: St. Martin's Press, 1998), chapter 34.
2. Julian Whitaker, M.D., and Brenda Adderly, *The Pain Relief Breakthrough* (New York: Plume, 1999).
3. Tantric *sutra* (or highly condensed telegraphic instruction) of the ancient tantric master Lord Shiva, elaborated upon in Osho's *The Book of Secrets,* chapter 71, sutra 98. *The Book of Secrets* explains Shiva's 112 tantric sutras. It was origianlly delivered as a series of talks, so Osho also answers questions from his audience about the sutras and about their experiences in meditation.

Chapter 5

1. Osho, *The Book of the Secrets,* chapter 68, question 4.
2. Ibid., chapter 67, sutra 95.

Chapter 7

1. Natalie Angier, *Woman: An Intimate Geography* (New York: Virago, 1999), 57–81. Includes an interesting chapter on the clitoris.
2. For a remarkable description of the twenty-two different parts of the intricately formed female genitalia, see Rufus C. Camphausen, *The Yoni: Sacred Symbol of Female Creative Power*, 96–103.
3. Nik Douglas and Penny Slinger, *Sexual Secrets: The Alchemy of Ecstasy*, 20th Anniversary Edition (Rochester, Vt.: Destiny Books, 2000), 148.
4. Another Shiva sutra included in Osho's *The Book of Secrets*, chapter 75, sutra 103.

Chapter 8

1. Another Shiva sutra included in Osho's *The Book of Secrets*, chapter 47, sutra 70.

Chapter 9

1. Osho, *My Way: The Way of the White Clouds* (Pune, India: Rebel Publishing House, 1995), chapter 6, question 1.
2. Mantak Chia, *Awakening Healing Energy through the Tao*, 32.

Chapter 10

1. Osho, *The Supreme Doctrine* (Pune, India: Rebel Publishing House, 1997), chapter 5, question 3.
2. Ibid.

Conclusion

1. Osho, *My Way: The Way of the White Clouds*, chapter 6, question 1.
2. Osho, *The Book of Secrets*, chapter 43.

Recommended Books and Resources

Books and Resources by Osho

The Book of Secrets. New York: St. Martin's Press, 1998.

My Way: the Way of the White Clouds. Pune, India: Rebel Publishing House, 1995.

Sex Matters: From Sex to Superconsciousness. New York: St. Martin's Press, 2003.

The Tantra Experience. Pune, India: Rebel Publishing House, 1998.

Tantra: The Supreme Understanding. Pune, India: Rebel Publishing House, 1998.

Tantric Transformation. Pune, India: Rebel Publishing House, 1998.

(For more information about Osho, visit www.osho.com, a comprehensive Web site in different languages featuring Osho's meditations, books, tapes, and selections from his talks)

Audiotapes and Books by Barry Long

Love Brings All to Life Audio Tapes

Making Love 1 & 2 Audio Tapes

Raising Children in Love Justice and Truth. London: Barry Long Books, 1998.

Stillness is the Way. London: Barry Long Books, 1989.

(Barry Long resource materials are available from: BCM. Box 876, London WC1N 3XX U.K: info@barrylong.org; www.barrylong.org; Valeo Resources, 2820 Sunlight Drive, Clinton, WA 98236, U.S.A. blf@whidbey.net)

Books on Sexuality

Angier, Natalie. *Woman: An Intimate Geography.* New York: Virago, 1999.

Camphausen, Rufus C. *The Yoni: Sacred Symbol of Female Creative Power.* Rochester, Vt.: Inner Traditions, 1996.

Chan, Jolan. *The Tao of Love and Sex: The Ancient Chinese Way to Ecstasy.* Hounslow, U.K.: Wildwood House, 1977.

Chia, Mantak. *Awaken Healing Energy through the Tao,* Santa Fe, N.M.: Aurora Press, 1983.

Chia, Mantak, and Maneewan Chia. *Healing Love through the Tao: Cultivating Female Sexual Energy.* New York: Healing Tao Books, 1986.

Douglas, Nik and Penny Slinger. *Sexual Secrets,* 20th Anniversary Edition. Rochester, Vt.: Destiny Books, 2000.

Richardson, Diana. *The Heart of Tantric Sex: A Unique Guide to Love and Sexual Fulfilment.* Arlesford, U.K.: 'O' Books 2002. (First published in 1999 as *The Love Keys: The Art of Ecstatic Sex.*) Translated into German, Spanish, Italian, French, Chinese. Excerpt and further information: www.love4couples.com. Available from oshoviha@oshoviha.org, www.oshoviha.org.

Books and Resources on the Sympto-Thermal Fertility Awareness Method

Fuller, Rose and Rev. J. Huneger. *A Couple's Guide to Fertility: The Complete Sympto-Thermal Method.* Portland, Oregon: Northwest Family Services, 1996. www.nwfs.org

Kippley, John F. and Sheila K. Kippley. *The Art of Natural Family Planning.* Cincinnati, Ohio: The Couple to Couple League International, 1997. See www.ccli.org

Weschler, Toni. *Taking Charge of Your Fertility: The Definitive Guide to Natural Birth Control, Pregnancy Achievement and Reproductive Health.* New York: Quill-HarperCollins, 1995. www.TCOYF.org

A new book is due out soon by the British Fertility Awareness Organisation. See www.fertilityuk.org for more information about its release.

If you would like to contact the sympto-thermal experts who contributed their expertise to the appendix, feel free to e-mail, phone, or fax them using the contact information provided below:

R. Harri Wettstein, PhD, MBA, MA, Director of Bioself SA, Geneva, Switzerland, www.bioself.com., and Secretary of SymptoTherm Foundation, Grand-Rue 41-CH-1110, Morges, Switzerland, e-mail info<@>symptotherm.ch, phone/fax +41 21 802 44 18, www.symptotherm.ch

Christine Bourgeois, President of SymptoTherm Foundation, 8 Sécheron, CH-1132 Lully, Switzerland, phone/fax +41 21 802 37 35, email c.bourgeois@swissonline.ch, symptotherm.ch, www.symptotherm.ch

"Making Love"
A Tantra Meditation Retreat for Couples

The author (also known as Puja) and her partner, Raja,
facilitate week-long meditation retreats and
guide couples into the art of tantra.

For further information and further communication:
www.love4couples.com
www.livinglove.com

Books of Related Interest

Tantric Secrets for Men
What Every Woman Will Want Her Man to Know
about Enhancing Sexual Ecstasy
by Kerry Riley with Diane Riley

Tantric Awakening
A Woman's Initiation into the Path of Ecstasy
by Valerie Brooks

The Sexual Teachings of the White Tigress
Secrets of the Female Taoist Masters
by Hsi Lai

Tantric Quest
An Encounter with Absolute Love
by Daniel Odier

Men's Business, Women's Business
The Spiritual Role of Gender in the World's Oldest Culture
by Hannah Rachel Bell

Sexual Reflexology
Activating the Taoist Points of Love
by Mantak Chia and WillIam U. Wei

Sexual Secrets: Twentieth Anniversary Edition
The Alchemy of Ecstasy
by Nik Douglas and Penny Slinger

The Complete Illustrated Kama Sutra
Edited by Lance Dane

Inner Traditions • Bear & Company
P.O. Box 388
Rochester, VT 05767
1-800-246-8648
www.InnerTraditions.com

Or contact your local bookseller